Young As You Look

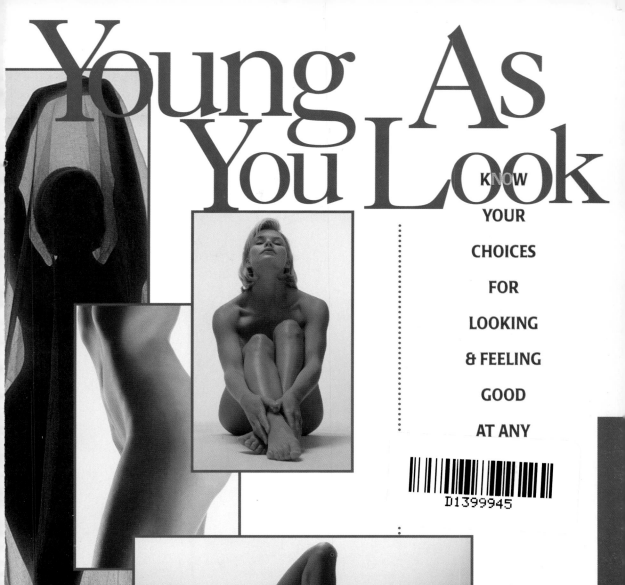

KNOW YOUR CHOICES FOR LOOKING & FEELING GOOD AT ANY

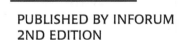

PUBLISHED BY INFORUM
2ND EDITION

DR. DON GROOT &
PATRICIA JOHNSTON

D1399945

InForum

Suite 207,

11523 - 100 Avenue

Edmonton, Alberta

Canada. T5K 0J8

(403) 488-6809

Web Site:

www.drgroot.ca

Designed

& Printed

in Canada by

Jang & Willson

Communications

ISBN 0-9696725-0-0

Contributors

Dr. Don Groot
Dermatologic Surgeon
The Dermatology and Laser Surgery Centre

Patricia Johnston
President, InForum

Dr. Martin Giuffre
Plastic Surgeon

Dr. Gerry Moysa
Plastic Surgeon

Dr. Howard V. Gimbel
Ophthalmologist
Gimbel Eye Centre

Dr. Harold Johnson
Ophthalmologist

Dr. Bernard Linke
Prosthodontist

Dr. John Evans
Dentist

Dr. Margaret Oseen
Exercise Physiologist

Simon Bennett
Fitness Consultant

Suzanne Gillespi
Registered Dietician

Wendy Matthison
Fashion Consultant

Nancy Brook
Editorial Consultant

Dedication

*This book
is dedicated
to our two sons,
who are the
embodiment of all
things wondrous
and beautiful
in youth.
It has been
our joy to share
family life with
these two loving
and free spirited
young men.*

Acknowledgments

The contributors to this book extend beyond those formally or individually listed. Perhaps our greatest inspiration has been our patients. They have given freely to this book in many ways. Without their friendship and our mutual respect, this book would have been neither conceived nor written.

Our family and friends have provided encouragement and shared joy at various stages of this work. We would like to particularly thank a group of women who provided us with advice and direction for the first edition of *Young As You Look*. Thank you *Annabel Bowlen, Barbara Keir, Nancy Lees, Lynn Odynsky, Ann Sather, Gail Glowicki, Cindy Benson* and *Cathy Cristall*.

We truly appreciate the creative flare which *Ron Scott*, the producer of the *Young As You Look* video, brought to this combined project. His insight, understanding and ideas were in tune with our own and it has been a pleasure working with him.

Will Jang's creative design and artistic structure has molded the second edition of this book.

We would also like to express our gratitude to *Dr. Martin Giuffre* and *Dr. Gerry Moysa* for their invaluable assistance as consultants in the field of plastic surgery.

Support for the **Young As You Look** book and video project has come from many people in affiliated areas of medicine. We would like to thank *Robert Lavoie, Richard MacKay, Sylvia* and *Lou Vogel, Dianne Kinnahan, Ray Hunt* and *Linda Casson* for their ongoing support and encouragement.

Wanda Hillary has dedicated many hours of her free time to reading the manuscript for technical errors. Her attention to detail and patience with last minute changes and revisions has contributed immensely to the quality of the second edition.

The Canadian Society of Dermatologic Surgery has endorsed the second edition of the **Young As You Look** book and the video. We thank the members of the Society for sharing our vision.

Medicine is an ongoing exchange of teaching and learning amongst professionals. Those we would like to particularly acknowledge are the people listed on the right sidebar.

DG/PJ

Drs. Lloyd Johnston
Jerry Groot
Jack Groot
John Evans
Henri Carle
Kent Remington
John Arlette
Tom McQueen
Stuart Maddin
Alan Dodd
Alastair Carruthers
John Dmytryshyn
Caudio di Lorenzo
David McLean
David Duffy
Al Behm
Bob Coupe
Roberta Ongley
Virginia Killby
Bill Wood
Shelly Pollack
Jeff Klein
Sterling Baker
Richard Fitzpatrick
Jeff Dover
Mitch Goldman
Alastair McLeod
John Mitchell
Janice Liao
Elizabeth McBurney
Larry Warshawski
Pat McElgunn
Gaston Dumais
Carol Layton
Henry Roenigk, Jr,
Larry David
Eric Eisenberg
Leon Goldman
Dick Gregory
John Yarbourgh, Jr.
Chris Janssen
Bill Hanke
Randy Chapman
Terry Carlyle
David (Joe) Vassos
Don Yu
Anthony Sneazwell
Lefter Mantse
Jean Carruthers
John Voorhees
and the late Bill Stewart
Ted Tromovitch
and Sam Stegman.

Table of Contents

Table of Contents

Table of Contents

Table of Contents

Table of Contents

Table of Contents

Table of Contents

The *Search for Youth & Vitality*

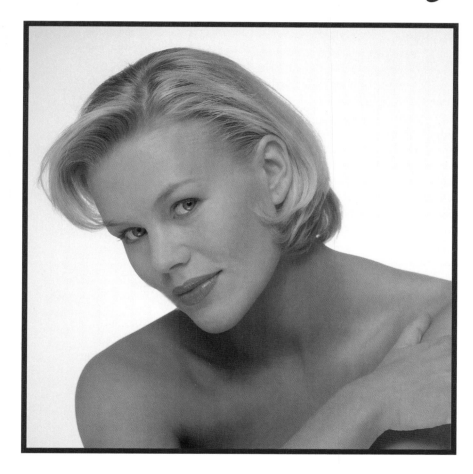

AN
AGE
OLD
PROCESS

*"What lies
behind us
and what
lies before us
are tiny
matters
compared to
what lies
within us."*

*OLIVER
WENDELL
HOLMES
M.D.
(1809 to 1894)*

INTRODUCTION

Many centuries ago, Aristotle observed that personal beauty is a greater recommendation than any letter of introduction. Little has changed since those ancient times.

A youthful appearance at any age will reflect and reinforce our feelings of inner vitality. Some of us are blessed with a genetic makeup which will keep us looking young and healthy throughout life, but the majority of us must help our bodies along.

Young As You Look is a book about the natural and medical alternatives for maintaining a youthful appearance at any age.

"All would live long, but none would be old."
BENJAMIN FRANKLIN

In the eighteenth century, Benjamin Franklin recognized the desire of people to live long, yet youthful and vital lives. Indeed, this search for youth dates back to at least the sixteenth century when Spanish explorer Juan Ponce de Leon set out on his search for the Fountain of Youth and instead found Florida. Throughout history and well into antiquity we find similar examples of man's desire to keep the ravages of time at bay.

Appearance affects our lives in many ways: relationships with others; feelings of self-confidence

and self-esteem; attraction to members of the opposite sex; and even success at work. "If you look good, you feel good, and if you feel good, you do good."

We believe that internal beauty is of greater importance than external beauty, yet in reality our external appearance is one of the vehicles through which we express our inner selves. We tell the world something about ourselves with our physical presentation: whether we are conservative or flamboyant, wealthy or poor, fit or out of shape.

Even if you put little emphasis on the way you look, you cannot avoid society's focus on external beauty through the media and a multitude of products and services. We are confronted daily with the media's view of the perfect woman or man. She, for example, is no less than 5 feet, 9 inches tall, long-limbed and slim, has great bone structure, a wonderful, healthy mane of hair, flawless skin, and the perfect smile. This is what we have to compare ourselves with! It's almost impossible to pick up a fashion magazine or to turn on the television set without seeing women or men flaunting their attributes.

Yes, there are near-perfect physical specimens among us, but the truth is that most of us do not look like the pictures we see. Most never will. Perfect we are not, but through a program of self-improvement which includes skin care, nutrition, exercise, cosmetic artistry, hair styling, fashion, and the use of medical technology, we can make the most of what we have.

There is a tendency when looking at these symbols of perfection, to assume they have access to professional assistance in looking their best at any age. Likely this is true. Few, however, realize that these same professional services, which include those of dermatologists, plastic surgeons, dental specialists, estheticians, stylists, nutritionists, and fitness consultants, are available in most North American cities. They are not unique to the fashion centres of New York or Los Angeles.

The decision to seek professional help comes to each of us in different ways and at different times. Anne is an example of a late bloomer. She is a 37-year-old woman who became aware that the passage of time was beginning to show on her skin a couple of years ago as she was completing her final year in a university graduate program. Anne is fair skinned and had spent much of her youth in the sun. She was not an avid "tanner" but loved to ride horses and hike in the mountains. Without protection from the sun, she frequently burned the skin on her face, neck, shoulders, and arms and, as a result, sun-induced damage began to manifest itself in her early thirties. Being busy with

school and a young family, she was relatively unconcerned with these changes. Her attitude changed when she was assigned to work with a younger group of students on a course project. The moment of truth came when one of her co-workers asked her how old she was. Thinking nothing of the question, Anne told them her age. There was a pause and then a meek response: "Oh, you don't look that old." Despite this weak attempt at making her feel better, Anne was shocked. She was perceived as "that old!"

She went home and took a hard look at herself. The signs of aging were definitely there. Deep furrows were etched into her forehead and between her brows. Her smile lines were there even when she wasn't smiling, and small, fine wrinkles had appeared along her upper lip and around her eyes. Her hair was limp and shapeless, and she had a tendency to throw on what was most handy from her closet in the morning.

Enough was enough! She embarked on a program of external self-improvement to match the effort she was putting into internal self-development.

She sought medical attention for her wrinkles and became diligent about the use of sunscreens, sunglasses, and sunhats. A trip to the hair dresser, an updating of her wardrobe, and regular exercise took care of the rest. She doesn't look

25, but she does look and feel her best. Her appearance now reflects her feelings of youthful vitality. In her own words: "I feel fortunate that so many options to keep me looking and feeling my best are available as I get older."

This type of experience is not unique to women. George is 42 years old and has been divorced for a couple of years. While dating a 28-year-old interior designer, he overheard her describing him to a friend: "Well he's smart, wears great clothes, and has a terrific body, but he's a bit older than I am. He's 42, but I don't think he would look so old if he wasn't going bald." George was aware that he was thinning on top but he had no idea Catherine thought he looked old because of it. At the dermatologist's office, he was relieved to find he wasn't the only man with such concerns and was pleased to discover there was something he could do about his baldness. First, he was going to apply topical minoxidil to the balding area, and if that didn't work, he could always opt for hair transplant surgery.

Knowing where to start is a concern many people have. Joan is 45 and teaches preschool. One day she was playing at the water table with some three-year-olds. After a time, her hands had become white and wrinkled from being in the water for so long. She commented to the group of children that

playing in the water had made her hands look tired and old. One of her students looked up at her and replied: "It makes your face look tired and old, too." Out of the mouths of babes! Although Joan was amused by this response, she was also taken aback. She had been relatively unaware of the signs of age creeping up on her face. The effects of time and years of unprotected sun exposure were becoming quite pronounced. On relating this story, she wondered where she could go for advice and the help she felt she needed. She was unaware of her options and where she should begin.

This book has been written for the Annes, Georges, and Joans of the world, women and men who want to know their options and where they can turn for help.

The reasons people seek professional help for their appearance are complex, with psychological and cultural components. It is beyond the scope of this book to discuss these factors. It is our aim to recognize rather than deny these trends in our society and to provide a comprehensive overview of the current sources of help so an individual can make wise and informed decisions.

What has surprised us in speaking with individuals who are concerned about the signs of aging, is the lack of information and the misconceptions surrounding current medical options. The information is available in abundance from a multitude of sources including magazines, brochures, and television, as well as professionals such as physicians, estheticians, and hair dressers. The problem is that the information is frequently contradictory or so scattered it is difficult for an individual to assimilate.

Young as You Look is a book for adults of any age who want to recapture or simply maintain a youthful appearance. It is a practical, essential guide to looking and feeling good so you can be your best in all you do. It is a book about choices.

Basic
Body Care

The *Skin*

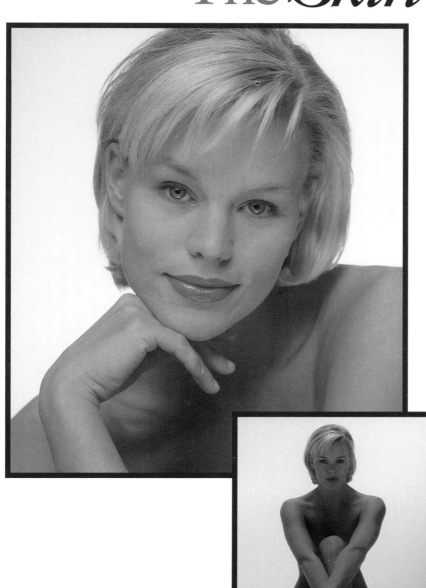

VITAL TO GOOD LOOKS

Making a good first impression is crucial; everyone knows that. While clothing, makeup, and hairstyle are all of importance, one of the first things people notice about you is your skin.

1 CHAPTER

O*ur agenda for the effects of time on the skin includes:*

▌ *skin structure*
▌ *changes with time*
▌ *changes in the skin*

We all have the potential for vitality, health, and attractiveness. The key lies in body care. Basic hygiene, nutrition, and exercise are essential ingredients to looking and feeling good. Yet, without a doubt, good looks begin with good skin.

The skin is more than just a bag in which the skeleton and organs are contained. In its own right, it is the body's largest organ. It is the interface between the body and an often hostile environment. The skin absorbs harmful external factors such as ionizing radiation, ultraviolet light, and hundreds of toxic fumes and chemicals, preventing them from entering the body and causing damage to vital organs. It monitors both internal and external temperature changes and adapts to these changes by sweating and through blood vessel dilation or contraction.

The skin reflects emotions, for example, the pallor of fear, the flush of excitement or anger, and the sweat of anxiety. It is also the organ most responsible for sexual attraction.

The skin reflects many internal diseases, acting as an early warning sign for such conditions as

diabetes, hormonal imbalance, and internal cancer.

The skin is unique. It differs from individual to individual and from race to race. It also differs dramatically from one area of the body to another.

Despite being unique in each individual, all skin has the same basic structure. It is made up of three layers: the epidermis, the dermis, and fat.

■ The epidermis is the outside or top layer of the skin, and is what you see when you look at the skin. The life cycle of the epidermis is about three weeks long. The bottom layer of the epidermis, which consists of new, rapidly growing cells, pushes up to replace the top layer of dead cells causing them to be sloughed off. The epidermis protects the skin and is very effective at blocking entry of foreign materials at the molecular level. Pigment cells are found in the epidermis and in the deeper layers of the skin around the oil glands and hair roots. The skin receives its color from pigment cells that produce melanin.

■ The dermis is the middle layer and contains the foundations or building blocks of the skin. The various components of the dermis are: elastin tissue (elastic protein) which gives the skin tone and makes it supple;

Elements of the Skin

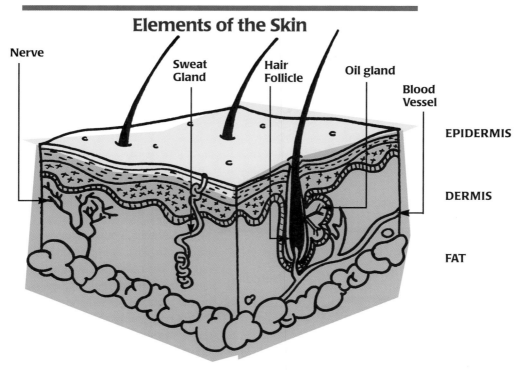

Nerve

Sweat Gland

Hair Follicle

Oil gland

Blood Vessel

EPIDERMIS

DERMIS

FAT

collagen (fibrous protein) to provide strength and structure; blood vessels which deliver essential nutrients and remove wastes; nerves which make the skin one of the most sensitive organs in the body; oil glands to lubricate the skin; and sweat glands which regulate fluctuations in body temperature. The dermis is the most vital part of our skin and is the layer where many signs of change are manifested.

■ A thin layer of fat is found underneath the dermis. It not only provides a protective padding, but also gives the skin a full, healthy look.

CHANGES WITH TIME

Our passage through time is marked by the celebration of our birthdays. This annual recording of our chronological age does not necessarily parallel our biological age. In fact we frequently compare an individual's chronological age to their biological age by such references, as she doesn't look that old or he certainly looks older than his years.

Time is only one of a number of the factors which determines our biological age. Heredity has a strong influence on the way in which we age, suggesting that our

CHAPTER 1

cells may be genetically pre-programmed to deteriorate or die according to a certain time-oriented schedule. This is known as the "alarm clock" theory of cellular aging.

Environmental factors place wear and tear on our cells contributing to their eventual deterioration. Where we live, the lifestyle we lead, our attitudes, and our access to modern medicine all

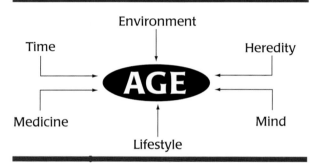

have positive or negative influences on the aging process depending on the choices we make in life.

The skin is one of the key indicators of our chronological and biological age. A wrinkled, sallow complexion suggests that a person is old and unhealthy, whereas a smooth, evenly colored complexion suggests youth and vitality. As we get older our skin passes through many transitions, some of which are influenced by our exposure to environmental factors.

Infancy: Infant skin is soft, pale, and vulnerable. The collagen in a baby's skin has not yet thickened and shows none of the brittleness that comes with age; it is very supple. The pigment cells are at a low level of activity producing little melanin. They have not yet been assaulted by ultraviolet light and are uniform in distribution, giving an even hue to a baby's skin.

Childhood: The skin is "learning" to adapt to the assault of the sun's rays as well as to other external abuses and stimuli. Although the skin's hue is still even, pigment irregularities and other changes, such as freckles, are beginning to appear. The collagen is shifting away from "baby type" suppleness to the more condensed and rigid "adult type" collagen. Blood vessels grow in response to the skin's nutritional needs, and dilated vessels may appear.

Adolescence: The skin is exposed to more external and internal stresses, such as sun, alcohol, drugs, and hormonal changes. Hormonal stimuli are causing a rebellion in the oil glands and hair roots. Acne and excess or decreased hair growth may result. Pigment cells are stimulated to give a rush of color in sexual areas and pigment spots of various types may appear. Changing body shape and rapid growth may cause stretch marks. The skin is becoming more adult-like and may soon be assaulted by the changes of pregnancy, birth control pills, sports trauma, and delayed reaction to excessive sun exposure and other toxins.

The Twenties: The skin has reached its developmental peak. It is supple and strong, and because hormonal equilibrium is relatively stable, problems with pimples and oiliness have abated.

The Thirties: The signs of aging begin to appear in most individuals. Damage due to sun exposure begins to manifest itself, particularly if an individual has been in the sun for many years without protection. Fine lines will appear around the eyes and mouth, and the skin may begin to lose some elasticity as the collagen in the dermis begins to clump up. With continuous exposure to the sun and internal hormonal changes, the pigment cells become less efficient at producing melanin, giving an unevenness of color. Silver streaks appear at the temples and thinning of scalp hair may occur in both men and women.

The Forties: The changes that began at 30 become more dramatic. Lines due to muscle pull, such as frown lines, laugh lines, and crow's feet, remain when the muscles relax. They are etched in the skin. Gravity begins to pull in areas where the skin has lost elasticity, causing it to sag. This is particularly true for the skin of the eyelids and around the jaw. The skin recovers less quickly from such abuses as fatigue, stress, and alcohol, partially because the circulatory system is no longer as efficient. Dark spots, often referred to as age spots, may appear. Hormonal change associated with menopause may lead to dry skin, excessive and unwanted hair in certain areas, thinning scalp hair, and a reduction of lubricating mucous in the vagina, eyes, and mouth. Recent studies suggest that testosterone decline in men as early as the forties is responsible for changes in the skin and hair growth patterns, as well as sexual desire. Hormone replacement therapy for men is 20 to 30 years behind that for women.

The Fifties Plus: The signs of aging, including fine and deep wrinkles, sagging skin, uneven color, and fat deposits are much more pronounced. The incidence of skin cancer and other age related blemishes is much higher. These signs will continue to develop unless something is done. The earlier the program of intervention, the less drastic it needs to be.

CHANGES IN THE SKIN

The changes that occur in the skin over time are manifested in different ways at different times. Conditions such as acne and wrinkles are well known signs of change.

Much can be done to prevent and correct these signs of change. These options have been discussed in detail throughout the book.

Acne

Acne is a condition in which the oil glands are unusually sensitive to the normal complement of hormones. Although acne can occur at any age, it is frequently associated with the teenage years when the skin tends to be hypersensitive to normal hormone levels.

Pimples develop when oil glands attempt to push the thick, buttery oil through tiny pore openings. The oil contains irritating substances that backfire into the surrounding tissue creating a mosaic of papules (red bumps), pustules, cysts, and blackheads. Subsequent scarring may ensue from damage to the skin's underlying architectural framework. Damage from severe acne to the architectural building blocks of the skin may actually make the skin susceptible to premature biological aging. For example, deep creases may appear between the nose and the corner of the mouth in the early twenties rather than in the forties.

Active acne can be devastating. In its aftermath, the acne prone person may be left physically and psychologically scarred. The key is prevention and early intervention through the help of a skin specialist. A variety of topical medications, which are applied directly to the skin may suffice for mild acne. More aggressive acne,

however, may require systemic medications such as Minocin (minocycline), a potent yet low risk antibiotic. This is taken by mouth in the form of a capsule. Such medications may be combined with regular treatments of ultraviolet light therapy, cortisone injections, and liquid nitrogen sprays. When acne is resistant to all other forms of treatment, a medication known as Accutane (isotretinoin) may be required. This derivative of vitamin A is a very potent medication which has some side effects, so the decision to use it is weighed carefully by the doctor in consultation with the patient.

Once acne scarring has occurred, a variety of resurfacing techniques, as well as collagen implant therapy, can be used to improve the appearance of the damaged skin.

Wrinkles

Wrinkles are simply folds and creases in the skin. Curses can be heard worldwide each morning as men and women inspect their faces in the mirror for this sign of aging. A number of factors contribute to the formation of wrinkles.

Heredity: We inherit a predisposition for the deterioration of the skin's building blocks, the fibrous protein known as collagen found in the dermis. If you look at your parents and grandparents, you will have a good idea of the pattern of

YOUNG AS YOU LOOK

wrinkling you might expect to see in yourself. Unfortunately, we cannot choose our ancestors so we cannot prevent this predisposition to wrinkling.

Sun Damage: Collagen deterioration is accelerated by the sun's rays. The Ultraviolet B (UVB) rays and the longer Ultraviolet A (UVA) rays of the sun both penetrate into the dermis, causing the breakdown of collagen and the formation of wrinkles, as well as other signs of sun damage: dilated superficial blood vessels; pigment changes; and scaly patches. If you travel to areas of the world such as California and Australia where the sun is intense and many people have fair skin, you may notice that many of them look older than their age. This is due to sun damage.

Muscle Pull: Consistent tension in a particular area of the face due to a habitual facial expression can result in a permanent furrow. Frown lines between the brows, fine lines around the eyes (better known as crow's feet), and smile lines extending between the nose and mouth are common examples of muscle pull furrows.

Gravity Changes: Young skin, because of its elasticity, can withstand gravitational pull. With age, degeneration of the collagen and elastin in the dermis makes the skin more susceptible to the pull of gravity causing it to sag. Droopy upper eyelids and bags under the eyes and jowls are common

examples of the impact gravity can have on the face. The "mirror test" shows you how gravity may have affected your facial aging. Lying on your back, hold up a mirror and examine your wrinkles looking at the depth of creases and angles over the bones. Now, lay the mirror flat on the table and gaze down into it. You will notice that certain areas of your skin are looser than others.

Hanging yourself upside down or yoga-like headstand exercises do not reverse the changes that gravity, day in and day out, etches in your face. It's simply too short a time to be effective. The same applies to gravity boots and inversion devices. The only result will be sore ankles and puffy eyes from fluid shifts to the loosely bound skin around them.

Sleep Creases: Vertical lines on the forehead and the cheeks can be caused by habitually pressing the face into a pillow night after night while sleeping. As the skin loses its elasticity it does not snap back in the morning and these lines become permanent. Sleeping on your back will prevent this problem but may cause sleepless nights for your partner if you tend to snore.

Fat Loss and Redistribution: Loss of the fat cushion or redistribution of this cushion in the third layer of the skin often occurs in the fourth to sixth decade of life. A redraping of the skin results, with furrows and creases appearing on the forehead, around the eyes,

Wrinkles

PHOTO
COURTESY OF
DR. DON GROOT

Wrinkles

Causes	Zone of Damage	Prevention	Rejuvenation
Heredity	Entire face & neck.	Oral Antioxidant: • Vitamin E • Vitamin C • Zinc (controversial)	Medicated Creams • Tretinoin • Alpha Hydroxy Acids Resurfacing • Laser Resurfacing • Chemical Peels • Dermabrasion Collagen Replacement
Sun Damage	Unprotected skin on the face & body.	Sunscreens, sunblocks, sunglasses, protective clothing.	Medicated Creams • Tretinoin • Alpha Hydroxy Acids Resurfacing • Laser Resurfacing • Chemical Peels • Dermabrasion Collagen Replacement

and on the chin and neck . The pull of gravity also comes into play because in certain areas the skin lacks the cushion-like support of the fat. The result is often a gaunt, wrinkled appearance.

In each individual these various components have a different impact. Generally, the degeneration we inherit establishes the foundation for the other factors. Sun damage clumps up the protein in the dermis, and with subsequent muscle pull, gravitational pull, sleep compression, fat loss and redistribution, the folds and creases take shape.

Wrinkles

Causes	Zone of Damage	Prevention	Rejuvenation
Muscle Pull	Forehead.	Avoid repetitive muscle pull, e.g. pursing lips to chew.	Laser Resurfacing
	Between eyebrows.		Collagen Replacement
	Between nose and corners of the mouth.		Brow Lift (forehead wrinkles)
	Around the lips.		Muscle Relaxing Injections • Botox
Fat Loss & Redistribution	Eyelids.	No practical prevention.	Facelift
	Cheeks.		Eyelid lift
	Jowls.		Brow lift
	Neck.		Tumescent Liposuction

Pigment or Color Changes

Hormonal imbalance and sun exposure can cause pigment changes which in turn cause irregularities in skin hue. Pigment irregularities can occur on any part of the body but tend to be worse in areas of sun exposure, such as the face, neck, upper chest, and hands.

Hormonal imbalance and variation in pigment cell sensitivities are commonly caused by oral contraceptives, pregnancy, and estrogen hormone supplementation. The result is a "mask of pregnancy", and blotchy discoloration of the skin. Sun exposure aggravates this problem and can be responsible for the development of pigment irregularities. Many treatments used for wrinkles due to sun damage, including medicated creams and resurfacing techniques, are also effective in evening out skin color (Chapters 6 and 7).

Vascular Changes in the Skin

Facial Veins: Facial veins, referred to medically as telangiectasia, are permanent dilations of the small, superficial blood vessels on the face. Chronic exposure to sun and wind are the most common causes of facial veins, although heredity also plays a role. Excessive, regular consumption of alcohol can cause facial veins, which adds a disturbing stigma to the condition. In some instances, facial veins may be associated with disease entities such as lupus erythematosus, dermatomyositis or rosacea. Hormonal imbalance caused by pregnancy or oral contraceptives may also result in the appearance of facial veins.

Cosmetically, facial veins, can be very disturbing. They change the color of the skin giving it a ruddy, weathered appearance. Fortunately, with the advent of target specific vascular lasers, facial veins are easily removed.

Birthmarks: Birthmarks occur when the body mistakenly distributes an excessive number of primitive vascular (red) or pigmented (brown) elements within the skin. Port wine stains are the most common type of vascular birthmarks, while pigmented birthmarks are less common. The variable pulse width (VPW) green or pulse dye lasers and the Q-switched ruby,

Alexandrite or Nd:Yag lasers have provided individuals with excellent treatment options which in the past were not available.

Cherry Angiomas: Benign blood vessel tumors known as cherry angiomas, may appear over the torso with age. They vary in size from tiny red dots about the size of a pin-prick to larger and thicker ones. They may appear in showers where 20 or 30 spots surface overnight. If cosmetically unacceptable, they can be removed simply and effectively with the VPW or pulse dye lasers.

Leg Veins: Spider veins is one of the many names for the small, superficial dilated veins that frequently occur on the legs. Telangiectasia is the medical term for these veins but they are also referred to as cosmetic veins, venous blemishes, venous blushes, vanity veins, venous sprays, sunbursts, or pregnancy veins. Spider veins frequently appear in women in their twenties, but can occur in later years as well. Treatment for spider veins is usually sought because they are cosmetically unacceptable not because they cause the individual discomfort or affect the body in any other way.

Some women are also predisposed to the dilation of larger, deeper veins, a condition commonly known as varicose veins. These can be distressing, particularly if they appear in large

YOUNG AS YOU LOOK

numbers. In addition, they frequently cause the legs to ache.

As with so many signs of aging, heredity is the major reason for problems with dilation of blood vessels in the legs, although they are aggravated by oral contraceptives, pregnancy, hormone therapies, trauma, high impact jogging and aerobics, and long periods of standing.

Sun exposure is frequently responsible for the appearance of small blood vessels on the face and upper chest, but is not usually responsible for leg veins.

Sclerotherapy is the treatment of choice for leg veins. It not only works for the majority of leg veins but it is also more cost effective than laser therapy. Although, very small veins with a blush-like appearance are best treated with the pulse dye laser and resistant, large, thick veins are responsive to the VPW laser (Chapter 7).

Redundant Skin

When elasticity is lost and the skin no longer responds to pulling or stretching by snapping back, the skin becomes redundant. The collagen and elastins in the dermal layer have become damaged due to sun exposure or have deteriorated due to a hereditary predisposition. The problem is further aggravated by the pull of gravity.

Excess skin can occur in many areas of the body including the face, the neck, the breasts, and the abdomen. Excessive weight gain causes the skin to be stretched for extended periods of time, and subsequent weight loss will often leave older skin sagging. An example of this is the crumpled-looking abdominal skin many women are left with after several pregnancies.

Little can be done to prevent redundant skin, however a variety of surgical techniques, such as facelifts, eyelid lifts, and tummy tucks, have provided relief for many women and men (Chapters 8,14).

Stretch Marks

Known medically as striae, stretch marks are the visible evidence that the skin's building blocks (collagen and elastin) could not keep up with its need for growth. Seen under a microscope, a stretch mark will reveal only a few elastic fibers in the center and an abundance of curled and clustered elastic fibers at the edges. The collagen fibers are separated rather than grouped in bundles.

Stretch marks are formed when the skin stretches at a rate that cannot be sustained by its elasticity. They may appear after rapid weight gain, spurts of growth, and pregnancy. The development of body contours, such as breasts or the bulking up of muscles, as seen in weight lifters, can also cause

1 CHAPTER

stretch marks. Anything that increases the body's cortisone levels, as is the case during puberty, obesity, weight gain, the injection of cortisone medications, or even the application of potent cortisone creams will increase the likelihood of stretch marks.

Stretch marks initially appear as red or purple lines of varying lengths and widths. Sometimes they are wrinkled and shiny. Gradually they fade to a color a shade lighter than the surrounding skin.

Women are more prone to stretch marks than men, and the marks usually appear on the breasts, the lower abdomen, the buttocks, and thighs. Men tend to get stretch marks only on the buttocks and outer thighs.

The regular use of tretinoin in high doses has provided the first effective treatment for this condition. Although, lasers, such as the Ultrapulse carbon dioxide laser or the pulse dye lasers, are beginning to make some inroads into the therapeutic options for stretch marks (Chapter 15).

Cellulite

Few skin problems are more mysterious and cosmetically aggravating to women than cellulite. Heredity plays a large role in determining whether or not a person will be plagued with cellulite, although other factors such as weight and muscle tone are important as well. Despite low body weight and good muscle tone, some people still have marked cellulite. Others are blessed with a wonderfully uniform fibrous collagen net that leaves the skin even and smooth.

The bumpy, puckered, and dimpled irregularities of fat collection which occur over so many women's buttocks, hips, and thighs are called cellulite. These areas are often the first to attract fat and the last to lose it. Men are less likely to have problems with cellulite because of differences in hormonal make up and in their pattern of fat distribution.

A mesh of collagen fiber holds the fat under the skin. The bumps, dimples, and accompanying shadows of cellulite are simply the fat pushing out of the holes in the mesh. In order to reduce cellulite, the amount of fat must be reduced, the supporting muscles must be toned up, and the surrounding and intertwining protein mesh work needs to be altered. Although cellulite is difficult to get rid of, a proper diet will reduce the fat, exercise will tone the underlying muscles, and vigorous massaging will break down the protein mesh work and the fat stores, helping to improve the appearance of this condition.

From a medical standpoint, topical aminophylline gel has been helpful for many people (Chapter 15).

Age Spots

Commonly known as "liver spots" (although they have nothing to do with the liver), age spots frequently occur on the torso, the back of the hands, the arms, and the face. These spots usually occur because of a hereditary predisposition to them, although they can be caused by sun damage. The sun also tends to accentuate existing spots. Age spots range in size from small freckle-like brown spots to larger flat, brown spots and raised, dry or greasy, brown bumps known as seborrhoeic keratoses.

Use of sunscreens can minimize the appearance of these spots. Without protection the sun will cause them to become darker than the surrounding skin.

Several techniques are available to remove age spots including bleaching creams, cryotherapy and removal with a Q-switched ruby, Alexandrite or Nd:Yag laser (Chapter 6 and 7).

Skin Tags

Small tags of excess skin can appear anywhere on the body but are most frequently found on the neck, in the armpit, under the breasts, and in the groin creases. They may become irritated with friction particularly in overweight people. When the skin is confused as to which direction it should grow, it simply grows out and skin tags appear. Medically, these tags are known as acrochordons. Avoiding excessive weight gain and constrictive clothing which causes friction, helps prevent skin tags from appearing. Skin tags can be easily removed by a dermatologist.

Skin Cancers

The incidence of skin cancer has increased significantly over the past few years. Sun exposure, particularly in fair skinned individuals, can cause skin cancer which should not be confused with the benign spots of aging. Any spot that peels, crusts, itches, hurts, changes color, suddenly appears, or cannot be identified as benign, should be assessed by a dermatologist. These signs may indicate a cancer. Fortunately, most skin cancer can be cured, particularly if recognized and treated early.

The *Skin*

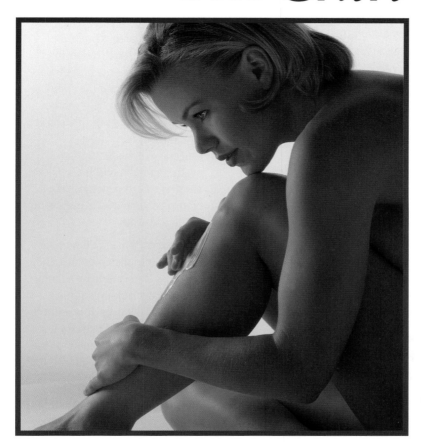

**TENDER
LOVING
CARE**

*A person's
skin says a
lot about
their
physical
health and
emotional
state, but
most neglect,
or through
lack of
under-
standing,
even
abuse it.*

CHAPTER 2

Our agenda for younger skin includes:

- *protection from the sun*
- *biofeedback*
- *alcohol and smoking*
- *stress*

A youthful appearance begins with prevention. Protecting yourself from the sun, controlling your muscle movements, and limiting your exposure to stress, smoking, and alcohol are of key importance in maintaining a youthful look to your skin. Sun protection is by far the best way to prevent wrinkles and other signs of aging such as loss of elasticity, pigment changes, altered skin texture, and dilated blood vessels.

PROTECTION FROM THE SUN

Sunlight is a time bomb. It tends to go off earlier in fair skinned people who have less intrinsic pigment protection. If you are in doubt about its impact on skin, try this test: look at the sun-protected areas of your body, such as the buttocks or breasts, and compare them to areas that have had a lot of sun exposure over the years, such as the V of your neck, your face, and the back of your hands. Notice the protected areas have none of the signs of aging that appear in the sun exposed areas: irregular pigmentation, wrinkling, and dilated blood vessels.

The Sun's Harmful Radiation

The sun emits three forms of radiation: infrared, visible, and ultraviolet. Infrared and visible light are valuable because they provide warmth and the ability to see. But ultraviolet light can be harmful. It consists of three basic wavelengths: Ultraviolet A (longest), Ultraviolet B (mid-length), and Ultraviolet C (shortest). Each penetrates the atmosphere and affects our health in different ways.

UVB Rays: Since UVB rays are absorbed into the epidermis, they can cause skin cancer by altering the normally well-organized behavior of the cells. It is as if the cells of the skin are panicking in response to the continuous abuse of the UVB rays.

The incidence of skin cancer doubles every 300 miles (485 km) we move closer to the equator.

The absorption of UVB rays in the epidermis also causes pigment cells to become less efficient and uniform in producing melanin. The demand for overtime production due to UVB rays results in inefficiencies and causes blotchy discoloration of the skin.

Not only are UVB rays absorbed into the epidermis, but they continue on through to the dermis. Here the UVB rays wreak havoc. By breaking down the collagen and elastin building blocks, they cause

CHAPTER 2

wrinkles; by clumping up the protein, UVB causes the skin to take on a thick leathery texture; and, by weakening the walls of small blood vessels, web-like lines known as spider veins form on the surface of the skin. These characteristics often do not appear for months, years, or even decades after the sun exposure.

The sun is not the only source of UVB light rays in our environment. The tungsten-halogen lamp, which is in common use in our offices and homes, transmits UVB rays through the protective quartz lining on the inside of the glass bulbs. The purpose of the quartz lining is to prevent the glass from melting because the energy emitted is very hot. However, the amount of UVB emitted from a 50 watt halogen lamp at a 25 centimeter distance can be equal to that emitted by the summer sun. To prevent this hazardous effect a UVB protected glass should be installed in front of the lamp.

UVA Rays: Recent research into the impact of UVA rays has shown this wavelength may be as harmful to skin as are the UVB rays. This is important to know since many suntan parlors use UVA wavelength bulbs. UVA is absorbed into the epidermis and passes through to the dermis. It does this much more efficiently and in much greater amounts than UVB rays. This realization has changed the "safe sun" rules.

- UVA rays are high in intensity all day long, and not just between 10 am and 2 pm as are the UVB rays.

- UVA rays are similar in intensity from one season to another, while UVB rays are less intense during the winter months.

- UVA rays are similar in intensity in any geographic location between the two poles whereas UVB rays become more intense as the equator is approached.

- Unlike UVB, UVA rays can penetrate through glass and plastic.

UVA and UVB rays can both be damaging to the eyes, as they are able to penetrate the protective covering of the eye known as the cornea. The resulting damage to the lens and the retina may cause cataracts and visual acuity problems. Since UVA rays pass through glass and plastic, many sunglasses are ineffective against them.

The sun also affects the immune system. UVB and, in particular, UVA rays can damage the Langerhans cells which are important components of the immune system within the skin. Their role is to recognize threats to the body in the form of viruses and other diseases. These cells then set the defence system in motion by instructing white cells, the soldiers of our immune system, to search and destroy. If the Langerhans cells are wounded, they become inefficient or ineffective in fulfilling their role. Ultraviolet light can damage white blood cells as well, rendering them impotent in the face of the enemy. The result is that cells normally held in check may be given an opportunity to grow uncontrollably as is the case with cancer. In addition, as damage to the Langerhans cells and the white cells reduces the overall effectiveness of the immune system, we may become more susceptible to viruses and other diseases.

UVC Rays: The impact of UVC rays is controlled by the ozone layer where these rays are absorbed. The small amounts of these rays that succeed in passing through the ozone layer are largely absorbed in the epidermis of the skin and do not penetrate to the dermis. Therefore, at this time, the effect of UVC rays is considered relatively inconsequential. One of the reasons for the concern over the gradual wearing away of the ozone layer, however, is that this wavelength of ultraviolet light could be very damaging to our overall health if received in larger doses. Perhaps this is one reason why the incidence of mole cancer has doubled in the last decade in North America.

Despite the potential damage the sun's rays can cause, ultraviolet light is a double-edged sword. Various wavelengths of ultraviolet light, in conjunction with medication, are effective in the treatment of acne, eczema, psoriasis, and other less common skin disorders. As with any potent treatment, the therapeutic use of ultraviolet light must be monitored carefully by a dermatologist in order to obtain maximum benefit with minimum risk.

Protection with Sunscreens

No doubt judicious and early use of sunscreens can protect against the most significant external factor in aging, the sun. Most sunscreens currently on the market, however, effectively block only UVB rays, not UVA. The concern is that people using high number sunscreens that block UVB rays may get high doses of UVA which can be very damaging to the skin. The natural warning signs, such as sunburn are, however, suppressed by sunscreens designed for UVB rays.

Recognition of the damaging effects of UVA rays has set the wheels in motion for the reformulation of sunscreens to more effectively block UVA rays as well. Sunscreens contain various agents which have been proven to protect against the rays of the sun. Para-aminobenzoic acid or PABA, PABA esters (glyceryl, padimate A, padimate O or octyl dimethyl PABA), and cinnamates are all agents which effectively protect against UVB rays. Benzophenones (oxybenzone, methoxybenzone, and sulfisobenzone) and Parsol 1789 are effective in protecting

Characteristics of UV Radiation

UVA	UVB	UVC
Longest wavelength.	Mid-range wavelength.	Shortest wavelength.
High intensity all day.	High intensity between 10 am and 2 pm.	Largely absorbed by the ozone layer.
Intensity is similar from season to season.	Intensity is reduced in winter months.	
Intensity is similar for all geographical areas between the two poles.	Intensity increases close to equator.	
Penetrates glass and plastic.	Does not penetrate glass and plastic.	
Penetrates the epidermis deep into the dermis.	Penetrates the epidermis deep into the dermis.	Absorbed in the epidermis.
Frequently touted to be safe but is not.	Known to be unsafe.	Very dangerous if it penetrates the ozone layer in large amounts.

against UVA rays. So to be totally protected, select a sunscreen with a combination of two of these agents, one for UVB rays and one for UVA.

Theoretically SPF (sun protection factor) simply means the factor of time greater than normal that it takes for ultraviolet light from the sun's rays to burn the skin. For example, if the unprotected skin burns in one minute, an SPF 15 sunscreen would allow 15 minutes of sun exposure before a sunburn will occur. An SPF greater than 15 provides diminishing returns.

Sunscreens come in different base preparations: creams, gels, lotions, sprays, and ointments. The choice is an individual one; some factors, however, are worth considering.

CHAPTER 2

- If an individual has a problem with acne, an alcohol base or one which will not occlude the pores would be the base to choose. (Ombrelle 15 lotion or Presun 15 Facial are suggestions.)

- If an individual has dry skin or is using tretinoin (Retin-A, Stieva-A, Retisol-A, Rejuva-A, Renova, Vitamin A Acid) which tends to dry the skin, a cream base may be the best choice (Ombrelle 15, or Photoplex are examples). Retisol-A is particularly good because it combines a broad base sunscreen with tretinoin and a moisturizer in a single cream.

- If an individual swims or participates in vigorous sports and perspires, sunscreens which will not wash off immediately are recommended. (Ombrelle 15 or Presun 29 are useful.) Note that occlusive and waterproof sunscreens may cause a sweat rash.

To select the sunscreen that best suits you, ask yourself the following questions:

- Does it protect my skin or do I have signs of sun exposure?

- Is it too occlusive and sticky?

- Do I break out in pimples when I use it?

- Do I break out in a rash?

Some advertisements recommend one type of sunscreen around the eyes, another for the lips, and so forth. It is better that you find one sunscreen that suits you and use it for all parts of your body. If you must subdivide the body, use one sunscreen for the face and another for the body; do not go beyond this or you may be discouraged from using a sunscreen at all.

When To Wear a Sunscreen

Since most ultraviolet damage is incidental and is not restricted to sunbathing, it is wrong to believe you do not need sunscreens simply because you do not sunbathe.

The need for sunscreens will vary with your skin, your activities, where you live, and your climatic conditions. For example, a fair skinned individual living in the southern United States should apply sunscreens several times a day. In northern Canada, however, daily use of sunscreens may be necessary only during the summer months or when taking part in outdoor winter sports such as skiing, skating, or tobogganing. Remember, ultraviolet light is reflected from sand, sun, water, snow, and ice. Remember, too, that a body immersed in water is not protected.

The frequency with which sunscreens should be applied varies with your activities. If you work in an office building all day, then an application first thing in the morning would be adequate. If you work out-of-doors, however, whether in winter or summer, several applications of high SPF sunscreens throughout the day would be necessary. You should remember that longer ultraviolet rays (UVA) can pass through glass. Broad spectrum sunscreens, therefore, should be worn if you spend a fair amount of time in the car or work close to a window during the day.

How To Apply a Sunscreen

The key to the effective use of sunscreens is to be diligent about their application. Apply them regularly and in adequate amounts. Thinly applied sunscreens markedly decrease the sun protection factor. Generally one ounce of sunscreen will be enough for one full-body application. If you are in the sun regularly and apply sunscreens properly, you should purchase a new bottle as often as you purchase toothpaste.

It takes practice and discipline. Not only should you be diligent about applying sunscreen to your own skin, you should be putting sunscreen on your children regularly as well. Make it a practice each morning to apply sunscreens to the exposed areas of their bodies before they dress.

Make the application of sunscreens a part of your daily skin care routine in the following way:

■ Cleanse the skin.

■ Apply sunscreens (minimum 15 SPF) to the areas of the body which will be exposed to the sun.

■ Apply a moisturizer if necessary, but note that some moisturizers have sunscreens in them; if a sunscreen has a lotion or cream base, it acts as a moisturizer.

■ Apply makeup.

■ Reapply as needed throughout the day depending on the amount of sun exposure and your rate of perspiration.

Sunscreens are most effective when they are applied to cool, dry skin so they should be put on 20 to 30 minutes before sun exposure. The reason for this is two fold. First, the sunscreen needs a cool, dry surface to bind to the top layer of the skin. Second, you are more likely to get a heat or sweat rash from the sunscreen if applied when the skin is hot because the sweat pores are open.

What To Do If You Forget Your Sunscreen

If you've been caught in the sun without sunscreen, you would normally expect to burn. A useful trick to prevent burning is to take acetylsalicylic acid (aspirin) before the burn appears. The first phase of a burn is largely the result of the ultraviolet light's interaction with the skin, causing the release of chemical prostaglandins. Aspirin is an antiprostaglandin, therefore it can effectively block the action of the prostaglandins in the skin if it is taken early enough. Two adult aspirin 3 times daily for 2 days may be helpful, if your digestive system can stand it.

Are Sunscreens Safe?

The safety of sunscreens has come into question. One concern is the sun's role in activating the body's vitamin D metabolism. Vitamin D is necessary to keep bones strong. The question is whether sunscreens inhibit the metabolism of vitamin D by blocking the sun's rays. In North America vitamin D is present as an additive in many foods. In addition, the amount of sun required to activate its metabolism is minimal – less than one hour of sun exposure per week to an area of the body as small as the palm of the hand. Even the most diligent users of sunscreen are likely to receive this amount of exposure on a weekly basis.

High SPF sunscreens have come into question recently because of the diminishing returns they provide as the SPF increases along with the potential problems that may be associated with them. The effectiveness of sunscreens dramatically increases from 45% blockage of UVB rays with SPF of 2 to 90% with an SPF of 10. The effectiveness tapers off to only an additional 5% UVB blockage with an SPF of 25 (95% effective) and little or no difference as one moves

into sunscreens with sun protection factors of 30 to 40.

Sunscreens that contain the PABA ester called padimate O (octyl dimethyl PABA) contain very tiny amounts of nitrosamine. Varieties of this nitrosamine have been found to be carcinogenic in animal studies. PABA-type nitrosamines, however, have not been used in these studies and absorption of sunscreens into the skin is minimal. Given these facts, it is unlikely the small amount of nitrosamine present in the sunscreen will do any harm. On the other hand, there is no real benefit in using higher concentrations of sunscreen with padimate O, such as an SPF of 40.

Allergic reactions can occur when applying any substance on the skin. Because the high numbered SPF sunscreens contain higher concentrations of active ingredients, irritation and/or allergic reactions are more likely to occur.

It is important to balance the issue of safety with the benefits offered by high SPF sunscreens. Remember, ultraviolet radiation is unhealthy and the more you protect yourself from it, the better off you will be in the long run. A sunscreen with an SPF of 15 which contains ingredients to protect against UVB and UVA radiation such as Ombrelle 15 is your best choice.

How To Be Safe In The Sun

■ Apply a broad spectrum sunscreen with an SPF of 15, such as Ombrelle 15, daily to sun exposed areas of the skin.

■ Apply the sunscreen about 30 minutes before sun exposure when the body is cool and dry so it will bind better to the skin.

■ Reapply sunscreen throughout the day according to the amount of sun exposure you receive. If you are participating in sports which make you perspire, reapply sunscreens every hour.

■ Protect the sun exposed areas of the body all year round.

■ Apply adequate amounts of sunscreen, one ounce for one body for one application. If you are using adequate amounts of sunscreen, you should be purchasing it as regularly as you purchase toothpaste. High-risk areas for cancer such as the face and hands should receive an extra dose of sunscreen. If you don't mind the look of a total block, use zinc oxide or titanium dioxide on the particularly sensitive areas such as the nose and cheek bones.

■ Be thorough in your application; sun exposed skin which is not covered will burn.

■ If you are wearing loosely woven clothing, put sunscreens on underneath them. The sun also penetrates wet clothing easily.

■ Wear waterproof or water-resistant sunscreens if you plan to be in the water. Waterproof sunscreens last for 1 1/2 hours and water-resistant sunscreens for about 30 to 40 minutes. They should be reapplied to dry skin allowing a bonding period of 20 minutes before re-entering the water.

■ Wear 100% UV-protected sunglasses that wrap around the eyes. Darker sunglasses do not necessarily filter out the UV rays unless they are specially coated.

Protection With Sun Blocks

Total sun blockage can be achieved by putting titanium dioxide on particularly vulnerable areas of the body such as the nose and cheeks. These products in their opaque form provide complete blockage from the sun's rays and the users can be identified by the war-like paint on their faces.

Recently it has been discovered that titanium dioxide of a

microscopic size of 10 to 50 nanometers is relatively transparent to visible light, but scatters ultraviolet light well, up to a sun protection factor of 15. In this form it becomes a sun screen rather than a sun block, for example PreSun 21 and Ombrelle 30 both contain titanium dioxide.

Melanin, the pigment our skin cells produce, has been added to creams to provide a good block for both UVA and UVB light rays. The creams are light to medium brown in color giving the skin a slightly darker hue when applied.

Protection With Glasses and Clothing

Sunglasses designed to reflect ultraviolet rays, will protect the delicate and thin skin around the eyes, as will broad-brimmed sun hats or visors. Wear them whenever you are in the sun. Look for sunglasses labelled "100% UV" protection and which have the designation "Z 80.3 Standard" on the temple piece or frame. This number means that the lenses meet or exceed the American National Standard Institute guidelines. Your ophthalmologist or optometrist can check your sunglasses for their ability to filter ultraviolet light. If your sunglasses do not filter UV light, they can be coated by an optometrist or optician to make them do so. Prescription glasses which are not sunglasses may also be UV protected.

Clothing may only partially filter ultraviolet light. Darker colors are not nearly as significant as the tightness of weave. Looser weaves allow the sun to penetrate and sunscreens should be worn under them. The sun will also penetrate wet clothes, so a waterproof sunscreen should be applied. Some clothing is now marketed with an SPF designation on the label.

TANNING

A tan signifies that the sun has damaged the skin to some degree. If you are applying a broad spectrum sunscreen with a SPF of 15 regularly, you should get a minimal tan or no tan at all.

At one time a tan signified wealth and health, but no longer! In fact, the deep, bronzed look is now "out", and companies which once promoted agents to enhance a tan are now actively promoting sunscreens.

Tanning Creams

If your motive for getting a tan is to have a so-called healthier hue, there are products available which will color your skin to look as though it is tanned, for example, Clarin's Self Tanning Milk, Estée Lauder Tanning Cream, and Lancôme Tanning Cream. Tanning creams contain dihydroxyacetone (DHA) which chemically reacts with the top layer of the skin to produce the appearance of a natural golden tan. This is a safe and effective way to achieve a summertime glow. After applying these creams, it will take a couple of hours for the color change to take place and it will last several days until the top layer of skin is gradually sloughed off. These products are much better than the skin colorants of the past which tended to streak the skin and stain clothing. Many tanning creams contain sunscreens and tanning accelerators, as well.

Some tanning agents, better termed coloring agents, can be taken orally. These agents contain carotenoids (cousins to carotene found in carrots) which are deposited in the fat and reach the epidermis through the sweat pores thus giving a tanned appearance. Some of these agents, unfortunately, may give a tan like color that has an unnaturally orange hue. Because the skin is thicker on the palms of the hands and the soles of the feet, these areas become distinctly orange in color when these agents are used.

Tan Accelerators

Tan accelerators, sometimes referred to as tan promoters, speed up the tanning process so the time of exposure to ultraviolet light is less. In some ways the principle is similar to that of the pre-holiday tan: the sooner you tan, the sooner

you willl be protected from a sunburn. This is true; tan accelerators, however, do not protect the dermis from damage which is partially responsible for premature aging and, to a lesser extent, skin cancer.

Psoralen is one active ingredient used in tan accelerators. It stimulates the pigment cells to produce more melanin when exposed to the sun. This results in the rapid development of a tan with less ultraviolet light exposure. Psoralen is extracted from citrus oil and other plant substances, and is found in such citrus fruit as limes. Even the juice from a lime, when applied to the skin, will tan that area faster than the surrounding skin.

Tyrosine is another ingredient sometimes added to tan accelerators to stimulate melanin production. It is a building block of the pigment protein melanin. Its usefulness for this purpose is not as well researched as psoralen.

Some tan accelerators also contain sunscreens to protect against burning. This, however, reduces the benefit of the tan accelerator in that it will take longer to get a tan because the sunscreen blocks ultraviolet light which interacts with the stimulator to produce melanin. The benefit of a tan accelerator over any other tanning method is that it requires less exposure to the damaging rays of ultraviolet light to get the tan.

If used cautiously, tan accelerators are probably safe to use. But, in reality, there is no safe way to tan. In order for the skin to tan, it must be exposed to ultraviolet radiation which is damaging to the skin in any amount.

Tanning Beds

Tanning beds were thought to be safer than sunlight for many years, but this is no longer is case. In fact, they emit far more of the longer wave UVA light rays than the sun does. Fifteen minutes of exposure to UVA in a tanning bed is equivalent to three days of sitting in the sun. The UVA rays penetrate deeper into the skin but do not cause superficial burning unless the skin is exposed to them for long periods of time. Continuous exposure to UVA light rays, however, contributes to the skin's premature aging, the development of skin cancers, the suppression of the immune system, and damage to the eyes. Lying in a tanning bed is much akin to setting a bomb to go off at a later date.

The belief that tans from suntan parlors will protect you from the burning rays of the sun has little substance. The protection offered by a preliminary tan would only be equivalent to an SPF of 2. If a tan is the goal, it is better to start with a high SPF broad spectrum sunscreen and decrease the number as the skin adapts to sun exposure. If you do not want a tan, continue

using the high SPF broad spectrum sunscreen.

BEYOND THE SUN

Biofeedback: Another preventive measure in the fight against wrinkles is biofeedback. This process teaches conscious awareness of previously unconscious actions, thus enabling behavior change. Biofeedback is particularly useful for preventing wrinkles caused by muscle pull and sleep creases.

Watch yourself in a mirror while talking on the phone or eating. You will be able to see those muscle pull lines which are acceptable and those which are not. Scowl, frown, and grimace lines are esthetically less acceptable than smile and laugh lines. By watching which expressions cause which lines, you can train yourself to stop using unattractive expressions.

For example, 36-year-old Gail, found the lines around her mouth to be very distressing. Her dermatologist informed her that upper lip wrinkles can be treated medically, but that they tend to recur because of muscle pull. She underwent a mild chemical peel and was given a regime of alpha hydroxy acid and tretinoin to apply to her face daily. In addition, she began to use biofeedback to recognize the kinds of behavior which caused wrinkles to form along her lip. She realized that

CHAPTER 2

several habits were contributing to these lines, such as her habit of pursing her lips while chewing and jogging. She stopped chewing gum and worked to change her chewing pattern during meals. She also put on a little grin to stretch out the upper lip while she jogged.

Biofeedback can also prevent compression creases on the face. These are characterized by vertical lines which do not follow normal facial contours. They are usually caused when people sleep with their face into the pillow at night. As time passes the lines do not fade away with the morning light. To avoid these creases, observe the way you sleep. If your head faces into the pillow, train yourself to sleep in a position where your face is away from the pillow. We "deep sleep" only a few hours each night. With training, some degree of conscious control can be exerted over the remaining hours, but it takes discipline.

What might help? A tennis ball in a sock pinned to your pyjamas can help in training nightly body positions. Where you pin the ball will depend on the position in which you sleep. For example, if you sleep on your stomach, pin the ball to the front of your pyjamas. A shaped pillow that fits into the nape of the neck also helps to encourage sleeping on the back.

In addition, the application of adhesive tape to wrinkled areas, such as crow's feet and the lower forehead, may help to limit facial movements while dreaming.

No matter what is written, you should never do facial exercises, because they may involve muscle pull which can actually cause wrinkles.

Alcohol: Limit the consumption of alcohol, as regular, excessive drinking may permanently affect the skin. Alcohol causes blood vessels to dilate. This constant stretching of the vessels can cause the walls to weaken and break, resulting in a blotchy redness to the skin and superficial spider-like veins.

Alcohol is very dehydrating. This is why numerous glasses of juice are necessary "the morning after". In an effort to combat the dehydrating effect of alcohol and to keep the vital organs well supplied with necessary fluids, the blood will borrow water from other tissue cells including those in the skin. This depletion of moisture in the skin emphasizes facial wrinkles.

Smoking: Smoking contributes to the aging process in two ways. By constantly pursing the lips to inhale the smoke, small wrinkles form around the mouth due to habitual muscle pull. Exposing the face to smoke on a regular basis also causes constriction of the skin's superficial blood vessels. This inhibits circulation, which is important to the nourishment and cleansing of the skin. It is for this reason, as well, that smokers are poor healers.

CHAPTER 2

Oral ingestion of vitamins A, C and E may protect against aging and the damaging effects of smoke. Vitamin A affects cell maturation and vitamin E and C act as antioxidants which reduce damaging by-products produced in aging cells. These vitamins may also be useful therapeutic agents for smokers and for those of us exposed to smog and other forms of pollution. The use of these supplements is controversial, although studies are now being conducted. Your best bet, in any event, is to stop smoking.

Stress: Stress is a complex phenomena which, like the sun, can be a double-edged sword. It may be protective and productive, but, left unchecked, may be destructive. To a certain extent, stress is the driving force behind creativity and accomplishment. "If you want something done, give it to a busy person." Too much stress, however, can result in counter-productive behavior such as insomnia, overeating, smoking, and drug abuse, including that of coffee and alcohol.

In response to stress, mediators such as adrenalin and hormones are released into the body. In the past, these stress mediators were dissipated through physical activity so emotion and mind worked together. Sedentary jobs and lifestyles have changed this to such an extent that these chemical mediators are no longer burned off

and, as a result, become destructive to the body.

The combination of counter-productive behavior and negative stress takes its toll. Weight gain, wrinkles due to muscle pull, a pallid skin hue, postural changes, chronic fatigue, and negative personality traits are some of the symptoms of chronic stress. You look and feel older.

Rather than giving in to negative behavior which will only accentuate the problem, seek to make a positive change. Exercise is an excellent means of dissipating stress and should be one of the first steps taken.

Develop a program of internal harmony. This may have many facets including emotional, spiritual and intellectual. The end result will be that you and those around you will feel better. An added benefit is that medical studies have confirmed that positive harmonious thoughts enhance your immune system, which ties into every aspect of our health.

Seek professional help if need be.

Xanthines: Avoid excess amounts xanthines (caffeine and theobromine) which are found in coffee, tea, colas, and chocolate. Xanthines dilate blood vessels and may accentuate a ruddy appearance.

The *Skin*

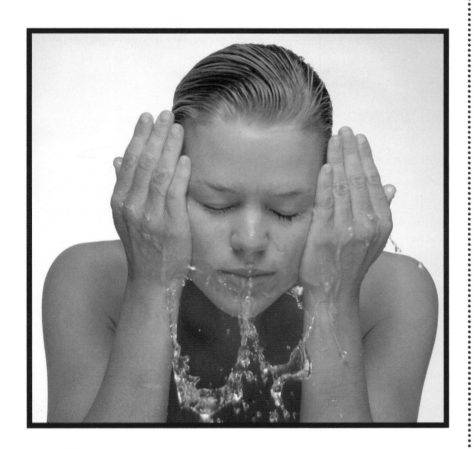

The cosmetic industry thrives on our desire to look and feel young and beautiful. It perpetuates myths about our need for skin care products in order to satisfy this desire.

CHAPTER 3

Makeup is the palette of the cosmetic artist. Features of beauty can be accentuated and less desirable features can be subdued. Artful application of makeup can greatly enhance ones natural beauty, yet when poorly applied it can be distracting.

Our agenda for beautifying the skin includes:

▌ skin care products
▌ makeup
▌ esthetic services

Cosmetics are a multi-billion dollar industry. As the "baby boom" generation ages, the industry has shifted its emphasis away from products for the younger generation to "anti-aging" products. Magazines are full of advertisements for products suggesting that they alone have the answer to aging. They would have you believe that the daily use of their product will assure you an everlastingly youthful appearance. Their claims, though seductive, are invalid.

Let's review the components of the skin. The skin has three layers: the epidermis (top layer), the dermis (middle layer), and the layer of cushioning fat (bottom layer). Aging largely affects the dermis and at this level a product must reverse the signs of aging to be as effective as it claims. At this time, most products are incapable of penetrating the epidermis and are therefore rendered relatively

impotent in their impact on aging.

On the horizon, however, are liposomes. These microballoons can carry active ingredients to deeper levels of the skin's surface. As cosmetic companies begin to use these microscopic vehicles to transport the active ingredients in their products, which they claim will prevent or reduce the signs of aging, to the dermis they will have to face the rigorous scrutiny of the Food and Drug Administration in the United States and the Health Protection Branch in Canada. This has two consequences:

First, if the product actually alters tissue, then it no longer is considered a cosmetic product. This means that the product must undergo scientific evaluation to support the claims, a very expensive process. If the claims are substantiated, the product may be reclassified as a drug, which means it will be shelved differently in stores. Depending on whether or not it is an over-the-counter or a prescription product, marketing strategies change.

Second, claims that are unsubstantiated risk being found to be fraudulent. The product could then be removed from the shelves without further warning. American law is more stringent on this point than is Canadian law.

These consequences apply to product claims whether liposomes are used or not. Most companies have chosen the simpler route of changing the anti-aging claims on their labels and in their advertisements. Others, however, ignore the warnings and continue to press their claims. It is up to you, the consumer, to evaluate these claims.

SKIN CARE PRODUCTS

Cleansers

Cleansing the body remains a basic and essential step in good grooming, affecting not only social interactions but, also dermatologic health. As with all skin care products, the problem lies in the choice of cleansers available. To be effective, a cleanser must remove the layer of dead cells on top of the skin as well as excess oil, makeup, bacteria and dirt. If a cleanser does not accomplish these basic functions, then problems such as acne, milia (tiny, hard, white cysts), and seborrhoea (scaly areas) are likely to develop.

Some individuals are under the misconception that these conditions can be treated with cleansers and a proper skin care regime. Unfortunately, this myth is frequently perpetuated by the cosmetic companies which sell skin care lines. The reality is that if a person has acne, milia or seborrhoea medical intervention is required. To counter the sensitivity of the skin to the body's hormones, people with acne usually require a medicated cream or antibiotics, such as tetracycline or minocycline

(Minocin) to control the formation of pimples.

Electrodesiccation is the treatment of choice for milia. The tiny, white cysts are destroyed with a mild electric pulse through a needle.

Seborrhoea is characterized by an inflamed flaking of the skin and an increase in oil production associated with an overgrowth of yeast spores. To treat this condition a mild cortisone salve or metronidazole (Metrogel) is applied to the inflamed skin and an oral medication called spironolactone (Aldactone) is taken to manage the excess oil production.

Many cleansers are available on the market today. They come in the form of soaps, creams, and lotions and each can be evaluated in terms of advantages and disadvantages and individual preference.

SOAPS

The two basic ingredients of soaps are vegetable fats and animal salts and these vary proportionally in the various soaps available. Other ingredients are frequently added to soaps for various purposes as well as to distinguish them from similar products. For example, some ingredients which may be added are deodorants and perfumes for body odor, abrasives for cleansing the pores, and oils such as coconut oil to make more lather.

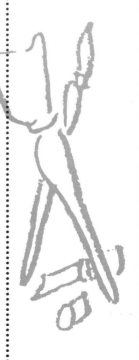

Soaps can be divided into four basic categories:

Bar Soaps: These soaps usually contain a relatively standard proportion of vegetable fats and animal salts. A popular example of this type of soap is Ivory. Sometimes, ingredients such as perfumes and deodorants are added which may irritate the skin. These soaps are now available in bar or liquid forms and generally clean the skin well.

Superfatted Soaps: The proportion of fat in these soaps is greater than in the bar soaps. As a result, these soaps may not clean adequately, in which case dead skin cells may build up, leaving scaly patches known as seborrhoea. A residual build up of oil may occlude the pores causing acne and milia. In some people, though, these soaps may leave the skin well cleansed yet soft and smooth. The choice of soaps, as with so many skin care products is a matter of experimentation and personal choice. Two commonly known examples of superfatted soaps are Camay and Dove.

Transparent Soaps: These soaps usually have a high fat content linked to glycerine or resin, and act in a similar fashion to the super-fatted soaps. An example is Neutrogena.

Detergent Soaps: Made from petroleum derivatives, detergent soaps contain synthetic detergents. They have an advantage over bar soaps when hard water is used, because the calcium and magnesium in hard water will react with a bar soap so a film of residue is left behind. This is not the case with detergent soaps. An example of a detergent soap is Lowilla.

ABRASIVE BARS AND CLEANSERS

Gritty, abrasive, and sandy cleansers are available in either bar or cream form and are becoming popular for two reasons. First, the cosmetic industry is targeting the male population because gritty cleansers appeal to the male image of tough-ness. Second, the concept of superficial self-sanding of the skin to supposedly freshen, smooth, and invigorate the skin, while removing the top layer of dead skin and any blackheads, appeals to both men and women. If this form of cleans-ing is too vigorous, however, it can cause irritation and subsequent irregular pigmentation. Further-more, in those people with acne, abrasives can rupture the weak oil glands and cause, rather than reduce, pimples. Overusing abrasive cleansers can also temporarily reduce the natural oil-and-water retaining components of the skin leaving it dry and dehydrated. If used gently, abrasive cleansers can give a rosy, shiny, and healthy appearance to the complexion by removing the top layer of dead skin cells, oil accumulation, and other facial debris. Even when used gently, abrasive cleansers may irritate and

CHAPTER 3

Skin Cleansers

Cleanser	Type	Example
Soaps	Bar Soaps:	
	• No Additives	Ivory
	• Deodorant	Irish Spring Dial
	• Perfumed	Estée Lauder Pierre Cardin
	Superfatted Soaps	Dove Camay Oilatum
	Transparent Soaps	Pears Neutrogena
	Detergent Soaps	Lowila
Creams & Lotions	Wipeable	Ponds Cold Cream
	Washable	Noxzema Cetaphil Cleanser

inflame the skin, causing tissue fluid to leak, swelling the skin, and making any wrinkles seem less obvious. This reaction is only temporary and may even be harmful.

CLEANSING CREAMS AND LOTIONS

Cream and lotion cleansers should not be confused with liquid soaps; they do not contain any soap. The oil in the cleanser dissolves greasy substances such as makeup and sebum on the skin's surface. The basic types of cream cleansers are those wiped away with tissue or those washed away with water.

Cream cleansers are useful for the removal of heavy or waterproof makeup and may benefit those with extremely dry skin and people who cannot tolerate regular or detergent soaps.

However, cream cleansers when used exclusively can promote dry skin because they do not remove the superficial layer of dead skin cells. The build up of these cells can result in a condition called seborrhoea which is often mistaken as dry skin. Blockage of the pores also promotes acne and milia.

Cetaphil cleanser is often recommended by dermatologists

as a cleanser for sensitive skin problems such as eczema.

Choosing the Right Cleanser

Mild soaps are better than creams. Finding the best soap to suit your skin type and your pocketbook is a matter of personal experimentation. The most expensive soaps, however, are not necessarily the best cleansers.

The cleanser you finally choose will depend on your skin type, how well the cleanser cleans your skin (no sticky or oily films), and whether the cleanser irritates your skin. You may wish to evaluate its smell, how long it lasts, and how much it costs. Your environment will also determine the type of cleanser you use; whether you are out-of-doors where it may be dry, humid, windy, sunny, hot, or cold, or whether you are indoors where heating systems, air conditioning, and fumes may have to be considered.

In general, cream and lotion cleansers should not be used except to remove heavy or waterproof makeup. Depending on the nature of your skin, you may choose one type of soap for your face and another for your body. Once again, this is a matter of personal choice.

Procedure for Cleansing The Skin

Wash your face twice a day with soap: once in the morning and again in the evening. Wash your body with soap once a day. If you have a tendency to dry skin, do not use soap over the whole body every day. Simply wash the areas that perspire: the armpits, the groin, and the feet. If a cleansing cream is necessary to remove heavy or waterproof makeup, wash away the oily residue with soap and water.

As to the amount of soap you use, let your environment be your guide. If the conditions in which you live are harsh and drying, it may be necessary to use less soap in combination with a moisturizer.

Assess yourself to determine if a moisturizer is necessary: wait 30 minutes after washing with soap, giving your skin the time it needs to replenish its natural oils. If your skin is dry after this, you probably need a moisturizer. You should apply it when the skin is moist. Be sure to repeat this test every so often, especially when your environment changes.

Be gentle! Scrubbing can cause irritation and will encourage the loss of your normal water-binding skin oils. Use lukewarm water. Avoid using hot water when washing both the face and body, as hot water encourages dryness. Detergent soaps are preferable to bar soaps if the water is hard. Bar soaps have a tendency to leave a gummy residue because the ingredients react with minerals in the water, leaving a residue on the skin as well as in the bath and sink.

Astringents and Toners

Astringents and toners are frequently used skin care products. Contrary to general belief, these products do not tone the skin. The reason the skin feels tighter after using astringents and toners is the active ingredient alcohol. Alcohol dissolves oil on the skin's surface and evaporates very quickly leaving a cool, refreshing, tight feeling after use. The use of plain soap and water twice a day, however, is as effective in controlling the build up of oil on the skin. Most people will find that astringents and toners are unnecessary and may actually dry the skin.

These products also contain ingredients such as colors and fragrances, which may cause allergic reactions. The only instance where astringents and toners might be recommended is in individuals with extremely oily skin. Even then they should not be used regularly. Intermittent spot application is usually all that is necessary.

Moisturizers

Three myths are associated with moisturizers and are frequently perpetuated by the companies promoting them. The first is that dry skin causes wrinkles, the second that moisturizers prevent wrinkles, and the third that all types of skin need moisturizers.

In reality, dry skin does not cause wrinkles. It is the top layer of the skin, or the epidermis, that is dry, whereas wrinkles occur in the second layer of the skin, the dermis. Moisturizers do not prevent wrinkles by counteracting dryness. Thus, the young girl in the ad who says she will fight aging all the way is using the wrong weapons if she hopes to win the battle.

Some moisturizers will reduce the appearance of fine wrinkles temporarily by retaining water within skin cells causing them to swell and erase fine wrinkles. Other moisturizers contain ingredients which irritate the skin. The inflammation causes the skin to swell slightly and this expansion stretches out the skin, reducing the appearance of existing wrinkles. Then there are moisturizers that contain ingredients that fill the furrows, giving them a smooth look. The length of time that these temporary wrinkle reducers last varies from only 3 hours to as long as 24 hours.

Special ingredients such as collagen, placental extracts, and vitamins are added to moisturizers but do not affect wrinkles because, at the molecular level, they are too large to be absorbed by the skin. In addition, if these products were actually successful in structurally repairing damaged skin, they would be subject to reclassification by the regulatory authorities and would not be sold at cosmetic counters. In fact, any hormones in moisturizers could potentially damage the skin and affect the body adversely through absorption.

Many companies are trying to jump on the tretinoin bandwagon by including vitamin A derivatives in their formulas, for example, vitamin A palmitate. The rationale is that enzymes in the skin will change the vitamin A palmitate into vitamin A acid or tretinoin, thus affecting the aging skin. In reality, only a very low dose of these vitamin A derivatives can be placed in these products, or the companies would likely become entangled with the FDA in the United States or the HPB in Canada. These low doses are unlikely to have any real impact on the skin. It is far better to obtain a prescription for tretinoin (Retin-A, Stieva-A, Rejuva-A, Renova or Vitamin A Acid) in an adequate dose, while using a moisturizer for any dryness caused by tretinoin. The other alternative is a product called Retisol-A which contains tretinoin in various concentrations, as well as a moisturizer and a broad spectrum sunscreen.

Glycolic acid and other alpha hydroxy acids have also been introduced into over the counter products. Some would argue that because these agents appear to alter the structure of the skin that they should be classified as medications. Be that as it may, they are available without a prescription and have been proven effective in reducing

fine wrinkles and evening out skin color. The deciding factors as to how effective these creams are would be the type of alpha hydroxy acid, the vehicle in which it is prepared, and the concentration. It is worthwhile to visit a dermatologist to find out which products containing alpha hydroxy acids are the most effective.

Tretinoin and alpha hydroxy acids are discussed in depth in Chapter 6.

Are Moisturizers Beneficial?

Moisturizers are useful for dry skin. The mechanism of action is to prevent the natural oils and water within the skin from escaping; they do not put moisture into the skin. This gives the skin a smooth, soft texture and, as mentioned, plumps up the fine wrinkles making them less obvious.

Chances are you will require a moisturizer at one time or another. Unless you have unusually dry skin, however, the use of a moisturizer should not necessarily become part of your daily routine. If moisturizers are used too often they can prevent the normal sloughing off of the top layer of dead skin cells. This gives the appearance of dryness and falsely induces the individual to use more moisturizer. This moisturizer induced dryness is called cosmetic seborrhoea. If the problem persists, the skin becomes inflamed, and scaly patches form.

YOUNG AS YOU LOOK

Choosing a Moisturizer

As with cleansers, the choice of moisturizers is a personal decision and involves a certain amount of experimentation to find the right one for you. There are three qualities to look for in a moisturizer: whether it helps control the dryness; whether it occludes the pores, which causes acne and milia; and whether it irritates the skin.

Oil and water are the two basic ingredients of moisturizers. The difference between moisturizing products is the ratio of these two ingredients in the products. Products labelled "oil free" may actually have oil in them, but the ratio of water to oil is usually much greater. Oils are necessary to trap the natural moisture. If you are unable to determine the ratio of oil to water in a moisturizer from its label, try the following tests before purchasing larger amounts of the product:

■ Put on some of the moisturizer. If the skin where you applied the moisturizer is warm, the moisturizer has a lot of oil in it; if the skin is cool, the moisturizer has a lot of water in it. The reason you can expect this reaction is that the water evaporates from the skin and evaporation is a cooling mechanism. Oil, on the other hand, does not evaporate. It traps the heat in our bodies.

■ Put a dab of moisturizer on a piece of tissue paper and hold it

over a hot light bulb for several minutes. If there is a lot of oil in the moisturizer, it will melt around the dab of moisturizer. The wider the spread of oil into the tissue, the greater the oil content in the moisturizer.

The essential difference between day, night, and eye creams is the ratio of oil to water. This is also the case for lotions, creams, and ointments. The body does not distinguish between day and night for its moisturizing requirements, and one type of cream will generally suffice for all moisturizing needs. For example, Moisturel is a very good overall moisturizer. We are psychologically conditioned, however, to distinguish between the moisturizing needs of the face versus the body. Many people would, therefore, find it difficult to put a body cream on their face or a face cream on their body. In addition, the pricing and packaging of moisturizers directs a customer to purchase one moisturizer for the face and another for the body. For example, body moisturizers often come in the form of lotions which make them easier to spread over a larger surface, and, generally, body moisturizers are less expensive.

Lotions tend to have a greater water to oil ratio and will allow the skin to breathe (sweat and cool) more than ointments which are often petroleum-based and greasy. Creams fall somewhere in the middle of the oil-to-water ratio.

CHAPTER 3

Beyond the two basic ingredients of oil and water, cosmetic companies try to differentiate their product from similar ones found at the cosmetic counters through creative packaging and by adding special ingredients for which they often make unsubstantiated claims. Here is a realistic look at some of the more commonly added ingredients.

■ Mineral oil and petroleum-based products are very good moisturizers because they effectively lock in the moisture. In high concentrations however they may occlude the pores, preventing natural oils from surfacing, resulting in acne and milia. They also tend to feel sticky on the skin.

■ Vegetable oils generally are not as effective for moisturizering as are animal fats and mineral oils.

■ Hormones and placental extracts attract and hold water, but can also cause allergic reactions. If these hormones are absorbed into the body, they may affect the internal organs.

■ Other ingredients, such as vitamin E, collagen, proteins, and amino acids may encourage skin hydration. They cannot, however, assist in rejuvenating aging skin because they do not pass through the top layer of the skin to the dermis where wrinkles originate. In addition, these ingredients can also cause allergic reactions.

■ Vitamin A derivatives have been added to some products as anti-aging agents. Whether or not the enzymes in the skin actually convert these derivatives into tretinoin, which is the rejuvenating factor in the anti-aging products Retin-A, Stieva-A, Retisol-A, Rejuva-A, Renova, and Vitamin A Acid, remains in question until they have been exposed to the cold light of scientific scrutiny. The doses are so low that even if they do convert to tretinoin in the skin, they probably do not provide the hoped for benefits. Examples of products containing vitamin A derivatives include Estée Lauder's Future Perfect Micro-Targeted Skin Gel, Prescriptives' Extra Firm, and Avon Bio Advance.

■ Chemical agents, such as urea, glycolic acid and lactic acid, improve the moisture retaining ability of the moisturizer. Examples are, Reversa lotion, Neo Strata cream, Lachydrin lotion, Lacticare lotion and Uremol lotion. These agents, often called "chemically-enhanced" moisturizers, are frequently recommended for dry skin problems and are most effective when put on moist skin. If they are not put on moist skin or are put on skin with small, dry skin cracks, they tend to sting.

YOUNG AS YOU LOOK

MAKEUP

Makeup is valuable for camouflaging the negative aspects of facial features and for highlighting positive features.

Allergic Reactions

Allergic reactions to makeup are usually due to such ingredients as perfumes, preservatives, antibacterial agents, and stabilizers. Perfumed products and perfume should not be used on sun exposed skin. The photo sensitizing agents that perfumes might contain can cause tenacious hyperpigmentation that leaves the skin looking brown and blotchy.

Cosmetic firms have improved their products significantly in order to prevent allergic reactions. It is in their best interest to do so and many of them have gone so far as to label their products "hypo-allergenic." But be warned: "hypo-allergenic" does not necessarily mean that the product will not cause acne; it may not even be less likely to cause irritation. Virtually all popular products are "hypo-allergenic", whether labelled so or not.

Another label you should be aware of is "dermatologist tested". This does not necessarily mean "dermatologist approved."

Cosmetic Artistry

Use of a cosmetic palette can fool the perceptions and create attractive visual illusions. Beauty-aid consultants can help with the art of cosmetic and hair styling techniques in order to camouflage or conceal imperfections. Women have an edge here since makeup, highlighting, shading, and versatility in hair styling is still within their realm, although this is gradually changing. Cosmetic artistry is the art of accentuating those features that, in our culture, we find attractive.

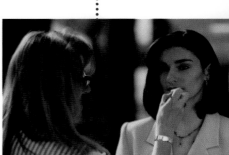

Proportion

The classically proportioned face for both men and women has balance. It is composed of three equal horizontal zones: from the top of the forehead to the eyebrows, the eyebrows to the bottom of the nose, and the nose to the bottom of the chin. Vertically, it is divided into five equal segments, each the width of the eye. Deviation from this need not be unattractive but these parameters provide a baseline from which to work.

The balance and harmony in makeup for a woman of 40 will be

CHAPTER 3

different than that for a 20-year-old. The colors you use, as well as the way in which you apply your makeup, must change as your facial features age. If makeup is applied correctly, it can minimize the signs of aging.

Through highlighting and shading, various features of the nose, cheekbone, jawline, chin, lips, and eyes can be accentuated or minimized. Areas of the face that are too narrow may be broadened by highlighting with lighter or brighter makeup. Areas which are too broad may be subdued by darker shading. Jowls or other areas of sagging skin can be de-emphasized by using a makeup twice as dark as the natural skin tone under the makeup base.

- **Foundations:** Foundations are effective in balancing skin texture and color. It is important, however, to select a product which does not cause such problems as acne, milia, or seborrhoea. Foundations come in three basic forms: water based, oil free and oil blend. Products which are water-based are generally best if your skin is aggravated by oily foundations, although they can be trickier to apply. A sheer base applied with a damp sponge is generally recommended by most cosmetic artists to obtain a natural look.

    Base makeups should be applied in such a way that the makeup will not gather in the creases, furrows, and wrinkles of the face as this will accentuate these problems. Concealers and cover-ups, properly applied under a base foundation, can help to minimize the impact of wrinkles. Dark colors cause fine lines to recede visually and to become less obvious, while lighter colors make them appear more prominent. On the other hand, deeper furrows and wrinkle creases may remain shadowed. Light-reflective highlighting creams and carefully feathered opaque covering creams can minimize the appearance of these creases.

- **Blush:** Rouges, if oil-based, can plug up pores, whereas powder blushes do not tend to cause skin problems. This is also the case with color products such as eye shadows, liners, and mascara. Blush highlights the attractive contours of the face and brightens a pale complexion. Powder, as a finishing touch over foundation, and blush will take the shine off the skin. This will serve to de-emphasize the shadows caused by creases and furrows. Loose, translucent powder is usually recommended, as it leaves a smooth finish and allows the underlying color of the skin to be seen.

- **Eye Makeup:** Eyes are a focal point and the way in which

Y O U N G   A S   Y O U   L O O K

makeup is applied can either draw attention to the signs of aging or subdue them. When selecting an eye shadow, choose a product which will not gather in the wrinkled skin of the eyelid; for example, pressed powder eye shadows versus creams. Matte colors are better than frosted shades because they do not accentuate redundant eyelid skin. Neutral, softer colors in shadows, eyeliners, and mascaras will add definition to the contour of eyes without emphasizing the signs of aging. Curling the eyelashes and defining the eyebrows will give a fresher, younger look to eyes.

If you wear glasses, take into consideration the effect the lenses have on your eyes as you apply your makeup. Glasses which correct nearsightedness make the eyes look small, whereas the opposite is true in the case of glasses which correct farsightedness.

■ **Lipstick:** The lips also change with time. They lose their definition as the dental structure changes and fine lines eventually appear around the lips from constant muscle pull. Lipstick tends to "bleed" into these creases, further accentuating these lines. To combat this problem with makeup, apply a moisturizing cream such as Elizabeth Arden's Lip Fix to the lips and surrounding skin before

applying your foundation. This will seal the fine lines, preventing the lipstick from bleeding. Add definition to your lips by using a solid lip liner along the natural outline of your lips, then apply matching lipstick to the entire surface of the lips.

■ **Permanent Coloration:** This process is similar to tattooing, where permanent color is imbedded into the skin to highlight lip lines and eyebrows, repigment areas of hypopigmentation, or soften the impact of scars. Allergic reactions to the dyes may occur, so test sites should be done before proceeding.

When colors are selected carefully and the technique is performed with sterility and a steady hand the results can be quite flattering. Unfortunately, there are no standards for training. It is wise to seek references and determine the level of training and experience of the operator.

The results are very difficult to reverse if an error is made or you do not like the outcome. Pigment removal lasers can be used to remove permanent makeup if it does not contain ferric oxide, which is common in permanent makeup preparations. Ferric oxide will turn black when exposed to laser light. A better alternative to

CHAPTER 3

Facials

	Heat Treatment (Steam, dry heat, sauna, lamps)	**Stimulators** (brushes, massagers, vibrators, electric probes)	**Masks** (clay, mud, moisturizing, exfoliating)
Stated purpose	• Deep skin cleansing.	• Close pores. • Reduce wrinkles. • Increase circulation.	• Close pores. • Reduce wrinkles.
What it actually accomplishes	• Softens the skin around the pores making it more pliable (blackheads may be removed more easily).	• Causes swelling and irritation which closes the pores and puffs up fine wrinkles for a few hours. • Stimulates skin circulation which may provide some subtle long-term benefits.	• Causes swelling and irritation which closes the pores and puffs up fine wrinkles for a few hours.
What it cannot do	• Does not help to drain pimples or remove milia because the openings to the pores are very small or non-existent.	• Does not prevent or reverse the signs of aging. • Does not tighten the pores; they cannot be tightened, as they have no muscles.	• Does not prevent or reverse the signs of aging.
Potential problems	• Aggravates acne and milia. • Blackheads reappear soon after removal.	• Aggravates acne and milia. • Warning: the electric needles can cause: • scarring • pigment changes • infection • transfer of disease.	• Aggravates acne and milia. • Causes contact dermatitis.

lasers is to introduce tannic acid into the unwanted color using a micropigmentation implant technique. This agent gradually bleaches out the mistake.

A note about the personnel at cosmetic counters:

They are there to sell cosmetics. As a rule, they cannot determine skin types, nor identify skin problems and how they should be corrected. The company they represent has trained them in techniques to market, apply and sell their specific cosmetic and skin care line. If you are troubled by your skin, see a dermatologist.

ESTHETIC SERVICES

Along with the rapidly growing cosmetic industry, the complimentary service industry in esthetics is on the increase. People visit their esthetician as often as once a week for manicures, pedicures, facials, removal of unwanted hair, tinting of eyebrows and eyelashes, and the application of makeup to enhance their natural beauty. Different techniques and equipment may be used to perform these services.

Manicures and pedicures are an excellent way to keep the hands and feet looking youthful and attractive. Removal of unwanted hair through waxing and electrolysis are alternatives to shaving in areas where shaving is not appropriate or does not leave a smooth hairless appearance. Eyebrow and eyelash tinting can add definition to these features and simplify the life of the individual who is always on the go. A word of warning, the dyes used for tinting may cause allergic reactions.

Facials are very popular. However, there is the frequent misconception that they are an effective way to treat complexion problems or aging skin. This is not the case. Facials can temporarily improve the texture and look of the skin. Medically sound alternatives are available to people who wish to control their acne or reduce the signs of aging. These have been discussed throughout the book.

A number of techniques are used to perform facials, including brushes and massagers, masks, heat treatments, vibrators, and electric stimulators. A realistic summary of the most common techniques for facials and what can be expected from them is provided in the table entitled FACIALS. In general, facials are not essential to good skin care. However, if you find facials relaxing and they make you feel good, go ahead and have them, as long as they do not irritate your skin.

Mild chemicals peels often referred to as acid washes are now being performed by many estheticians. These peels temporarily even out skin color and puff up fine wrinkles. The long term benefit of these treatments is in question, but many women swear by them. As long as an esthetician is properly trained and is using an acceptable level of concentration given that he or she has no medical background, the risks of permanent skin damage such as scarring are relatively low. It is important, however, to be aware that a chemical burn can occur.

The training and experience of estheticians varies immensely, therefore it is wise to be selective. Some estheticians have been trained in-house by another staff member, while others have received training at a cosmetology school. The training programs at these schools can also vary from a six week to a two year course.

Word of mouth is a fairly reliable means of finding a qualified esthetician, but always be prepared to judge for yourself. Ask about training and experience. Request references. If procedures which can be potentially damaging to your skin, such as electrolysis or mild chemical peels, are to be used, ask the esthetician to do a small test site so you can observe their technique and the results before proceeding with a larger area. Remember some areas of the body such as the upper lip scar more readily than others.

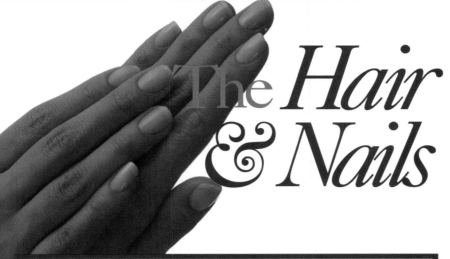

The *Hair & Nails*

**LOOK
YOUR
BEST**

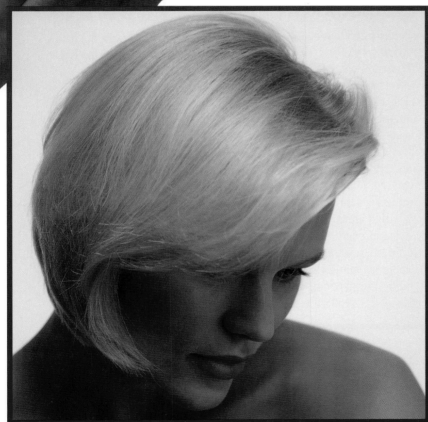

*Your hair
and nails
are both
important
contributors
to your total
look, and
given the
right care
they can
make you
look great.
On the other
hand, if
neglected,
they can
detract
from your
appearance.*

CHAPTER 4

Our agenda for your hair and nails includes:

▪ *hair today and tomorrow*
▪ *hair care*
▪ *nail care*
▪ *nail care products*

HAIR TODAY...
AND TOMORROW

Despite the important role of hair in protecting you from your environment (cold, heat, the sun's rays), you are probably most aware of its impact on your appearance. Social norms dictate how much hair is acceptable and where it is acceptable on the body. For instance, short hair may be in style one year and out the next. The hair care industry is thriving and it brings with it annual trends in hair styles and hair care products. In North America today, it is not acceptable for women to have hair in the armpits or on the legs, whereas in the 1960's this trend

was partially reversed, as the style of the day focussed on the natural look. Men with hairy chests are considered masculine but even this is subject to socially acceptable limits.

Hair is an integral part of the structure of your skin and, like your skin, it changes with the passage of time. A single strand of hair is made of several components: the hair shaft (the visible part of the hair) is dead; the hair follicle (sac) and the portion of the hair below the skin's surface is a single structure which lives and grows at an average rate of 1 to 3 centimeters (1/2 to 1 inch) per month. The hair follicle is an appendage of the epidermis of the skin. It extends into the dermis, from which it receives its blood supply and sensitivity through the surrounding network of nerves.

Hair develops in three phases: a growing phase, a transition phase, and a resting phase during which the hair is shed. On average it takes

A Single Strand of Hair

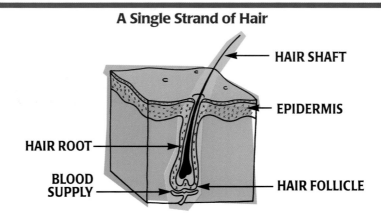

HAIR SHAFT

EPIDERMIS

HAIR ROOT

BLOOD
SUPPLY

HAIR FOLLICLE

a single scalp hair one to two years to pass through all three developmental phases. Although you shed hair every day, it grows back at about the same rate as you lose it. An adult has an average of about 100,000 head hairs and they are lost and replaced at a rate of approximately 100 hairs a day, under normal conditions. Hence the hairs which are found on the shower floor and tangled in hair brushes each day. Hair also tends to grow faster in the summer than in the winter.

Hair varies from individual to individual in color, texture, and amount. Redheads tend to have fewer hairs than do brunettes or blondes, but their hair is much coarser in texture. Blondes, on the other hand, have finer hair but lots of it. Brunettes fall somewhere between blondes and redheads.

Hair changes in color and amount with age. These changes can be distressing because they are highly visible signs of aging. They occur both in men and women but the norms of acceptability differ for each sex. For example, greying hair tends to be more acceptable in men than in women. Superfluous or unwanted hair is of particular concern to women, since hair on the face, around the nipples, and above the pubis is generally considered to be unacceptable. Hair loss is more apparent in men because it is regional, whereas in women it is more diffuse.

There are really no measures to prevent greying, growth of superfluous hair, and balding when they are associated with aging and when there is a hereditary predisposition for these problems. The medical options available to cope with excess hair and balding are discussed in Chapter 12.

Greying Hair

Greying hair is one of the most obvious indicators of aging, but is quite easily camouflaged by coloring the hair. Although grey is the color most often associated with aging, darkening of the hair is also a subtle indicator, particularly for people with fair hair. It is seldom that a blonde child retains a white head of hair throughout life. For this reason, many fair-haired individuals bleach and color their hair as they get older; they wish to retain the hair color of their youth.

With age, pigment cells throughout the skin and hair are lost. Hence the new hair growth is grey. The oft heard comment "I am going grey", reflects this gradual process. With advancing age, the grey hair is eventually replaced by hair which is totally deplete of pigment cells and is white in color.

Whether or not hair turns grey, and to what extent, is generally determined by hereditary factors. There are some rare conditions in which the body perceives the pigment cells in the hair as foreign and attacks them, resulting in loss of color unexpectedly at an early age. This can sometimes be brought on rapidly after a period of great stress, such as a terrible tragedy.

Superfluous Hair

In some women, age can cause hair to grow on the chin or upper lip, around the nipples, the breast cleavage, and above the pubic area. Many women, particularly in North America, find this hair unacceptable and seek to have it removed. One out of three women in North America does something for facial hair.

The majority of women with superfluous hair have no obvious underlying medical reason for this problem. It is usually the result of a hereditary predisposition. For example, excess hair is commonly seen in people of Mediterranean and Semitic descent and much less often in people from Northern Europe. Circumstances other than heredity, such as certain types of drugs, the overproduction of male hormones (androgens), or a hypersensitivity to normal amounts of these hormones may also account for unwanted hair.

The options for the removal of unwanted hair are many and varied and have been discussed in detail in Chapter 12. The most recent and significant breakthrough has

been the use of lasers for hair removal. Although still in its infancy as a method of hair removal, lasers promise to replace more traditional techniques, such as electrolysis, in providing a solution to unwanted hair.

Hair Loss

Hair loss associated with the aging process brings to mind balding men, but hair loss is not exclusive to the male gender. Women also experience hair loss with aging, but the pattern of loss is different. It tends to be less regional and more diffuse over the scalp. Women virtually never become bald from this process, but sometimes the hair can become very thin, particularly if there is a strong family history of male-pattern hair loss. Men, on the other hand, tend to lose hair initially at the temples and on the crown of the head. With time, the pattern of loss spreads from these regions until, in some men, a large portion of the head is bald.

Two factors contribute to hair loss associated with the aging process. One is heredity. With age, there is a genetic predisposition for hair loss, and this determines when, if ever, hair loss will begin. It is like an alarm clock which is set for different times in different people. This accounts for the wide variation in hair loss among people. Some begin to lose hair in their teens while others may never experience hair loss.

The second factor contributing to hair loss with age is hormonal sensitivity. With age, the hair follicle becomes hypersensitive to the normal levels of the male hormone androgen. This inhibits hair growth resulting in smaller, thinner hair as it passes through its developmental phases. Eventually, the hair becomes so small that it does not grow beyond the surface of the skin, giving the appearance of balding. The hair root is still viable and for this reason, male-pattern baldness has been responsive to the drug minoxidil (Rogaine, Minoxigaine or Apogaine). It is not the hormones which are out of sync but rather the hair follicle which is too sensitive to the normal level of hormones.

Other common causes of hair loss unrelated to age are categorized as external and internal.

External Factors:

External damage to the hair or skin can be caused by the rubbing of clothing such as helmets and protective equipment; bleaches, dyes, and permanent curl solutions for the hair; tight hair styles which compromise the blood supply to the hair root; and hair care utensils, such as tight curlers, which pull or tear at the hair. External damage can usually be corrected simply by avoiding those factors which cause the problem.

Internal Factors:

Internal causes include certain medications or drug therapies, such as chemotherapy for cancer, malnutrition, hormonal changes during pregnancy, iron deficiency, thyroid imbalance, and stress.

Internal causes must be identified before corrective measures can be taken. In some cases treating the internal cause will restore the normal growth of hair. If the hair does not grow back, then the use of topical minoxidil or hair transplant surgery can be tried, although the outlook is not always positive.

If sudden, extensive hair loss occurs, medical attention should be sought immediately, as the underlying cause may be serious.

Misconceptions:

Misconceptions about hair loss are many, and it is time to dispel some of these myths:

- Shampooing the hair frequently does not encourage balding. It simply removes those hairs that are ready to fall out. Excessive towelling or brushing and some hair care products may cause hair breakage which can mimic hair loss.

- Dandruff (seborrhoeic dermatitis) does not cause balding, although cleansing away the scale in an area of balding seems to allow the fine hairs that were trapped under

CHAPTER 4

the scaly skin to surface. This fine, fuzz-like hair does not tend to grow into longer, more mature hair.

■ Changing an already well balanced diet by eating more of one type of food, such as vegetables, will not stop hair loss associated with aging. Only in cases where diets are significantly deficient in a specific element such as zinc or iron will diffuse hair loss occur. Such a condition may also unmask male-pattern hair loss earlier in individuals who are predisposed to it.

■ Male-pattern hair loss may be inherited from either parent, not just the father. In some families, generations may be skipped.

■ Balding is not caused by wearing hats. The blood supply to the scalp is so extensive that any constriction that may occur from wearing headgear does not cause the problem. Hats, however, may result in breakage of the hair at the scalp, which gives a bald appearance.

HAIR CARE

Many hair care products are available and each affects the hair in different ways. When you cleanse or treat hair in any way, you are dealing with the hair shaft, that part of the hair which is visible and dead.

Shampoos

Shampoos are to hair as soaps are to skin; they are an essential part of good grooming. To be effective they must strip the hair of dirt and excess oil, while at the same time cleansing the scalp to remove the top layer of dead skin cells. The hair must be left undamaged and looking lustrous. Many shampoos do little to cleanse the hair but may beautify it.

Shampoos contain one or more of the following types of ingredients:

Soaps: Shampoos that contain soaps as the active cleansing ingredient may leave a residue on the hair if used in combination with hard water, thus leaving the hair dull. The residue, however, is easily removed with mildly acidic solutions such as dilute lemon juice. If the shampoo you use seems to leave your hair dull, it may be worthwhile to switch. Generally, more expensive shampoos are made with synthetic detergents which do not present the same problems as do soap-based shampoos.

Synthetic Detergents: Shampoos made with synthetic detergents do not leave a residue on the hair because they do not interact with hard water. The strength of either soaps or synthetic detergents, and to a lesser extent the amount of oils or conditioners present, determines whether shampoos are designated for dry, normal, or oily hair.

Acid: Many shampoos are alkaline in nature and can leave the hair looking dull and lifeless. To balance this effect, mild acids are added to many shampoos, hence the term "pH-balanced."

Conditioners: The purpose of a conditioner in a shampoo is to replenish the oils that detergents remove and to make the shampooing process more convenient. Shampoos that contain detergents and conditioners, counteract one another to some extent. This may reduce the overall effectiveness of the product.

Medications: Some shampoos contain ingredients which treat skin problems on the scalp. Dandruff is the most common of these conditions, and ranges in severity from a dry, flaky scalp to a condition in which the skin grows too fast and the oil glands become inflamed (seborrhoea). As dandruff becomes more severe, the scalp may become annoyingly itchy. Medicated shampoos contain agents which slow the growth of the skin and bring the inflammation of the oil glands under control, relieving the itch. They do not encourage hair growth. By releasing the tiny hairs trapped under the scaly skin, the hair may appear to be temporarily thicker. There is, however, no evidence that this fuzz-like hair grows to maturity and fills in areas of hair loss.

Conditioners

Conditioners are a particularly beneficial adjunct to cleansing the hair with shampoo because they reduce the trauma of combing the hair when wet and squeaky clean. They also contain ingredients which help to temporarily mend damaged hair by binding ruffled hair and split ends. This type of damage is often seen in hair which has been exposed to too much sun, has been colored or permed frequently, or has been subjected to chlorine in swimming pools. The active ingredients in these conditioners are proteins. Conditioners also contain quaternary compounds which help to control fly-away hair, a common problem in dry, cold climates and air conditioned rooms. The oils in conditioners help to replenish those which have been stripped from the hair in the cleansing process.

Not everyone needs a conditioner. Those who do not may find that the conditioner leaves the hair limp and oily looking. The decision as to whether or not a conditioner is necessary, and which conditioner to use, is one of personal experimentation and choice.

Coloring the Hair

Coloring grey hair may have a major effect on people's perception of age. Take, for instance, Janice, a

CHAPTER 4

38-year-old university professor who took a sabbatical. On her return, an acquaintance remarked that the trip had obviously done wonders for her because she looked ten years younger. In reality, though, Janice had taken the opportunity of her absence to dye her hair, covering up the significant amount of grey she had before she left.

Hair color preparations range from temporary coloring agents, which simply coat the hair with color, to permanent coloring agents, which actually penetrate the hair. The temporary dyes do not irritate the scalp or damage the hair, whereas permanent dying or bleaching of the hair may cause both problems. Semipermanent dyes offer a reasonable compromise because they last longer than temporary dyes, but are less likely to irritate the skin or damage the hair.

Although tradition says women color their hair and men do not, men are frequenting hair salons more often to have their hair color enhanced.

Mousses, Gels, and Hair Sprays

Hair mousses and gels are popular because they are good styling and holding solutions. They can, however, aggravate acne and milia on the face and neck, particularly in areas the hair touches, such as the forehead, cheeks, and the back of the neck. Allergic reactions to the ingredients in these products can also occur.

Hair sprays may also cause allergic reactions and have been reported to cause irritation to the eyes, respiratory problems, and even irregular heart beats. When using hair spray the face should be protected, in particular the eyes, and care should be taken to not inhale the mist.

NAIL CARE

Nails provide a protective covering to the ends of toes and fingers and are useful for manipulating small objects. They are also a symbol of beauty.

Each nail is composed of a root (or matrix), a body, and an edge. The root is concealed within a fold of skin, the body is the exposed portion attached to the surface of the skin, and the edge is that portion free of the underlying skin. The body and edge make up the hardened nail plate. New cells evolve from the root and from under the body of the nail. As these die, they become part of the hardened nail plate which is rich in calcium and a fibrous protein known as keratin.

The rate of nail growth varies. It is greater in the fingernails than the toenails, in the summer than the winter, and in children than in adults. Nails of individual fingers

Elements of the Nail

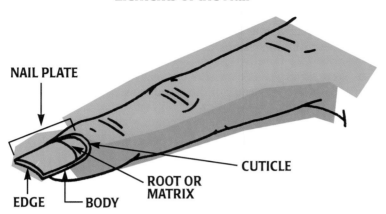

NAIL PLATE

CUTICLE

ROOT OR MATRIX

EDGE   **BODY**

on the same hand grow at different rates. The average thumbnail, for example, grows its full length within 4 to 6 months at a rate of 0.1 millimeter per day.

In children the nail plate is thin and pink due to the extensive network of blood vessels beneath it. Over time, the nail plate loses its transparency leaving an opaque white hue. Longitudinal ridges commonly appear on the nail after the age of fifty. Nails also tend to become brittle because their natural oils and moisture have been depleted. Exposing nails to harsh environmental factors such as detergents, as well as the use of various nail care products, simply adds to the problem.

Beyond the changes which occur over time, the condition of your nails tells much about the condition of your body. Spoon-shaped fingernails, for example, may suggest iron deficiency and its

accompanying anemia. Small red or brown linear streaks beneath the nails, known as splinter hemorrhages, may appear after trauma and are seen in conjunction with liver disease, heart valve dysfunction, blood poisoning, and scurvy. Clubbed nails, a condition in which finger tips appear bulbous, are seen with a variety of internal problems including lung cancer, and diseases of the liver, heart, and bowel. Paired white parallel bands across the nails indicate low blood protein levels. Half-and-half nails which are white near the roots and red at the tips are seen in people with kidney failure. Nails that lift up from their beds may be associated with thyroid abnormalities. Longitudinally ridged and fragmented nails may suggest abnormal functioning of the hypoparathyroid glands or poor circulation. If any unexplained condition of your nails appears, you should consult a dermatologist.

CHAPTER 4

Hand and Nail Care: DOs

■ Wear rubber gloves lined with cotton when your hands are in contact with harsh soaps, detergents or chemicals.

■ Wear gloves when doing work that might damage the hands or nails, such as gardening or shovelling snow.

■ After washing your hands, pat dry and, while moist, use a moisturizer on the hands, cuticles and nails. Chemically enhanced moisturizers that contain urea or lactic acid are even more efficient in binding water to the skin (Uremol, Calmurid, Lachydrin, Lacticare).

■ If your hands must be in and out of water frequently, apply a silicone or a similarly based protectant film that sheds water over the hands and nails (Prevex, Atrixo, Barriere Cream).

■ If nails darken despite good cleansing habits, a drop of lemon oil massaged twice weekly into the nail plate may work but must not be overdone or irritation of the surrounding skin and drying of the nail plate may occur.

■ Nail polish protects the nail from stains, physical trauma, and acts as a barrier to chemicals. Use it but don't overuse it or it may stain and dry nails, particularly if nail polish hardeners are used frequently. A base coat will allow your polish to last longer.

■ If your nails are dry, soak them for 10 minutes twice daily in warm water, pat dry and immediately apply one of the chemically enhanced moisturizers that contain urea, lactic acid or glycerin oil.

■ Sculpt and shape your nails by filing in one direction with a very fine file. Avoid vigorous up and down or back and forth motions which may tear apart the various layers of the nails. Avoid sharp angles. Attend to small cracks, snags and breaks immediately.

■ Treat yourself to a weekly manicure if possible; it is relaxing and keeps the nails healthy looking and attractive. Do not forget your toenails!

■ As they age, the nails thicken, grow more slowly, repair poorly and are susceptible to various skin diseases. Watch for changes and see your dermatologist early enough to treat problems.

Hand and Nail Care: DO NOTs

- Avoid digging blindly into a drawer or purse where a sharp object may crack or break the nail or harm the delicate skin around the nail.

- Avoid using the nails to do pick-up tasks. Use the soft ends of the fingers rather that the fragile nail; they will soon chip and break if used this way.

- Avoid gluing on false or molded nails; allergic and painful reactions may occur. "Mending paper" or tea-bag paper can be used to bridge large cracks.

- Do not reapply nail hardener or polish more often than necessary; these agents can discolor nails and make them brittle if overused. Try to repair your manicure rather than replace it. Avoid chipping and peeling off nail polish.

- Do not bother adding gelatin and calcium supplements to an otherwise well-balanced diet. They have no know positive effects on the nails despite certain claims.

- Do not use too much nail polish remover. Apply moisturizers after using nail polish remover in order to minimize the irritating and drying cation of the acetone.

- Do not grow excessively long nails; they are too prone to breakage.

- Wrapping nails is laborious and is difficult to do without help. Avoid this technique unless your nails are particularly prone to breaking.

- Do not push back your cuticles too vigorously or you will harm the growing moon of the nail. Push them back only when the skin around the nails is warms and wet and therefore softer and easier to manipulate.

- Avoid applying sharp instruments under the nails. They might break the nail to skin bond.

- Do not ignore nails that separate from their beds (it may be due to iron or thyroid deficiency), nails that thicken (it may be fungus infection) or pit (it may be psoriasis). See your doctor. The nail and skin reflect internal well being or disturbance.

CHAPTER 4

An astute observer could deduce more about your state of health by careful examination of the nails, hair, and skin than even you may know from living within your own body.

Nail Care Products

Preventive measures to protect your nails should be taken and these have been listed in the tables on *Hand and Nail Care: DOs and DO NOTs.*

Nail care products can enhance the appearance of your hands and feet, yet at the same time they are harsh and may damage the nails over time.

Nail Polishes

Nail polishes have been promoted as beautifiers, hardeners, and protectors. They beautify the nails by coloring them and have become a fashion accessory. Most polishes have similar chemical ingredients; nitrocellulose and resins are used to provide glossy, hard finishes. Polishes do not actually strengthen the nail. Some contain ingredients, such as nylon, which make the polish itself stronger.

Nail polishes contain ingredients that can be very irritating to the skin and may cause allergic reactions. For this reason it is advisable not to touch the skin until the polish has adequately dried (at least two hours). If you are in a hurry, try putting your freshly polished nails under cold running water for 3 to 5 minutes. This hardens the polish quickly.

Nail Polish Removers

Nail polish removers are not good for your nails. In order to effectively remove nail polish, strong solvents are used such as acetone, which leach oil and moisture from the nails leaving them hard and brittle. This is the case even with removers containing conditioners or oils.

Nail polish removers may also be very irritating to the skin. Avoid contact with other parts of your body, particularly the face, when using nail polish removers and wash your hands thoroughly afterwards. Try to control the amount of remover you use by touching up your nail polish rather than removing and reapplying new coats.

Nail Hardeners

Nail hardeners may do more damage than good. Although they harden the nails, they may also irritate the skin around the nail, discolor the nail, cause the nail to detach from the nail bed, and may even cause hemorrhaging under the nail.

Cuticle Removers

The cuticle protects the root of the nail from which our nails grow and should not be removed. For this reason, the use of cuticle removers is not recommended. They also contain very strong alkaline chemicals which are extremely irritating to the skin. The cuticles may be trimmed to avoid hang nails and to keep the hands looking well groomed.

Nail Creams and Cuticle Softeners

These products are essentially the same as moisturizers. Some of them are chemically enhanced with urea but otherwise they are not unique. Regular use of a hand cream, such as Norwegian Hand Formula will serve the same purpose.

Fitness

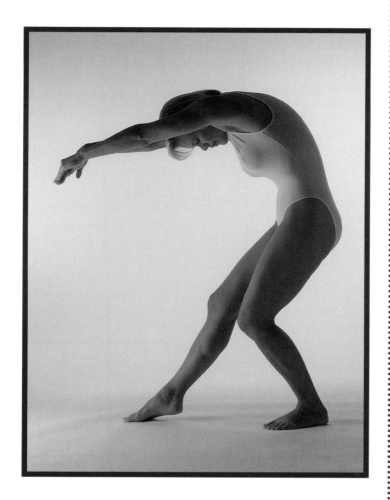

KEY TO HEALTH

Your lifestyle dictates how you appear to others. A balanced diet, adequate sleep, and a good exercise program, tailored to your schedule and your conditioning, are the best things you can do to keep yourself looking and feeling terrific.

CHAPTER

5

O*ur agenda for simplified basic body care includes:*

▋ *nutrition*
▋ *exercise*

Our lifestyle ultimately determines our health and the degree to which our bodies age. Individuals who are under stress, who do not get a sufficient amount of sleep, who lack proper nutrition and who live sedentary lifestyles are unfit, unhealthy and are susceptible to premature aging and disease. This results in suboptimal appearance and functioning. The body becomes biologically older than what is optimal for its chronological age.

The purpose of this chapter is to provide you with accurate information regarding the benefits and importance of a lifestyle which includes exercise and proper nutrition. However, if it is your desire to look better, to feel better, and to live a healthier life, you will need more than information and knowledge. You will need to make a commitment to change your way of living for the duration of your life.

NUTRITION

The fuel we provide our bodies is essential to life. Good nutrition is more than just eating well. It is a balance between healthy enjoyable eating, an active lifestyle, and self acceptance.

These three dimensions of life have a powerful impact on our health, our level of stress, and our energy levels. When these interact and are in balance with one another, individuals are free from psychological and physical illness and disease.

Self Acceptance

We cannot change our genetics and will have great difficulty changing what the society we live in has deemed as beautiful and healthy. Yet as individuals we can make a

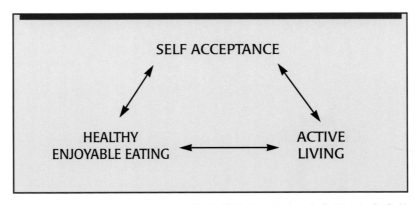

SELF ACCEPTANCE

HEALTHY
ENJOYABLE EATING

ACTIVE
LIVING

CH**APTER**
5

commitment to do the best we can with the cards we were dealt.

Naturally when we are eating well and getting regular physical exercise we feel better about ourselves. The increased self-esteem results in a more nurturing care of the body and this cycle soon becomes a lifestyle shift. It is in this balance that individuals take the best care of their bodies and their health. Ultimately the benefit is an increased sense of wellness. On the flip side we can easily recognize that when feelings of self acceptance are low, individuals may either overeat or undereat. This in turn impacts on any realistic goals of physical activity. Either lethargy sets in and the individual does nothing, or they become exercise anorexics.

By taking care of ourselves we can be our best self and in so doing we will feel good about ourselves, which in turn will encourage positive feelings and self acceptance.

Healthy Enjoyable Eating

Eating must be healthy to insure adequacy of nutrients and energy. It must also be enjoyable. When the enjoyment of eating is lost, individuals suffer from automatic eating, binging, and deprivation cycles.

What we eat has a major impact on how we look..."you are what you eat." If you undernourish your body with inadequate energy,

nutrients and water, you will appear listless, tired and pale. However, receiving enough calories, carbohydrates, protein, fat and water in a balanced regular diet will allow you to appear and feel energized, rested, and vibrant.

It is so easy to eliminate whole food groups, as trends often go. Or allow your body to become deficient in key nutrients, as the signs of neglect are easily disguised initially. In the long run, however, the body will manifest the effects and it may be too late to reverse the damage. A lifetime of deficient nutrition may result in such ailments as hypoglycemia, adult onset diabetes, heart disease, high blood pressure, liver disease, kidney failure and some cancers.

Active Living

Food is essential to life. Proper nutrition is essential to an energetic life. The uptake and utilization of glucose is essential to provide the energy we need for our regular daily physical activity. Glucose is the body's most efficient and preferred form of fuel.

Where can you turn for help in developing an optimal eating plan for yourself?

There is much contradictory and scientifically refutable information about nutrition. Many poorly controlled, so-called scientific studies, make claims that are unsupported, and either

CHAPTER 5

through ignorance or vested interest mislead consumers.

Each individual must take responsibility for sifting through the facts and the fallacies. Whenever claims are made about diet and nutrition determine whether the information is reliable or not.

Unreliable:

- Claims made without scientific research to back them up.

- Distortion of recognized nutritional facts.

- Recommendation of miracle foods or supplements as a cure all.

- Elimination of entire food groups.

- Recommendations for the use of only certain types of food.

- Promises of quick easy results.

- Emphasis on personal testimonies.

- Lack of professional credentials.

Reliable:

- Scientifically supported double blind studies.

- Credible source of information such as a registered dietician.

- Current research.

- All the facts are presented.

- No appeal to the emotions.

- Absence of sales pitch.

- Emphasis on a balanced diet.

- Information sources listed.

There is no danger in exploring alternative foods, natural foods, herbs, or vegetarianism, however insure your dietary intake remains nutritionally adequate and balanced. Consult a trained professional and be wary of individuals calling themselves nutritionists, this is a term almost anybody can use. A Registered Dietician has five years of training, including a University degree and an internship at a recognized hospital.

Nutritional Guidelines

Recommended Nutrient Intake (RNI) and Recommended Dietary Allowances (RDA) are guidelines established by the governments of Canada and the United States, respectively, through extensive research by the scientific community and health professionals. The recommended amounts of food in these guides will satisfy the eating requirements for 97.5% of the population for maintaining optimal health, free from disease. The Canada Food Guide and/or the Food Pyramid are practical tools which have translated these nutritional requirements into food groups.

The cornerstones of these guidelines which will provide for optimal nutrient and energy intakes include:

- eating a variety of foods from all four food groups:

  Breads and Cereals
  Fruit and Vegetables
  Milk and Milk Products
  Meat, Fish, Poultry
  and Alternatives.

- meeting your energy requirements for an active lifestyle.

- limiting fat intake.

- eating regularly and consistently.

- drinking adequate amounts of water.

Essential Nutrients

The body requires more than 50 essential nutrients per day. There is no substitute for a balanced diet in order to achieve these nutrients which can be divided into macro and micronutrients.

Macronutrients

Carbohydrates

Carbohydrates are oxidized to provide glucose to all the tissues in the body. It is necessary to obtain at least 50-55% of our daily calories as carbohydrates so that this readily available fuel is converted to energy as needed. Carbohydrates are found in the Breads and Cereals and the Fruit and Vegetable food groups.

Although choosing foods from these groups is recommended,

moderation is still key. Simply, if there is too much glucose in the blood stream the surplus is converted and stored as fat in adipose tissue.

The breads and cereals selected should be "complex", that is high in fiber and low in fat. Fruit should be fresh with seeds and skin intact and vegetables should be cooked minimally. Use these foods to respond to your energy demands in small amounts frequently through out the day.

If choices of carbohydrates are too simple such as refined cookies, chips, candy, sweets, and even juice, the sugar (glucose) is so simple that it is quickly absorbed and the body stores it as fat. The more complex and fiber rich a food, the slower the rate of glucose absorbtion and the more satisfying and beneficial the food is to the body.

The illustrated comparison of 100 calories of apple juice versus 100 calories of an unpeeled apple shows how the slow steady release of glucose through complex carbohydrates allows for the efficient, long lasting utilization of the fuel, whereas simple carbohydrates provide a quick fix of our energy needs. The inefficiency with which simple carbohydrates are used results in the excess being stored as fat.

Protein

Unlike carbohydrates, proteins are not used to meet the immediate

CHAPTER 5

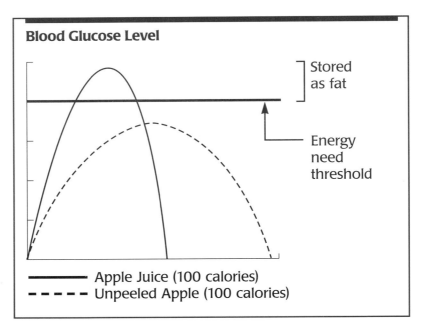

Blood Glucose Level

Stored as fat

Energy need threshold

——— Apple Juice (100 calories)
- - - - Unpeeled Apple (100 calories)

energy needs of the body as they are not absorbed for 1 to 3 hours after ingestion. They are important to the building and maintenance of tissue. The average adult needs about 0.8 grams of protein per kilogram of body weight daily.

The Milk and Milk Products food group is an important source of protein as well as carbohydrates and essential nutrients such as calcium, iron, and amino acids. The recommended adult consumption is two servings of this food group per day.

Food chosen from the Meat, Fish, Poultry and Alternatives group are likewise an important source of protein. Recommended servings would translate into 4 to 6 ounces of meat (of any origin) per day.

Protein foods can be high in fat content. Therefore it is important to select low fat Milk and Milk Products and unprocessed lean meats, as well as preparing these foods using low fat techniques. Choosing fish and seafood at least twice a week is recommended, as they contain no saturated fat and they provide a good source of polyunsaturated fatty-acids which have been shown to prevent heart disease.

Fat

Limiting fat in our diets is essential because it plays a primary role in problems of heart disease, diabetes, and some cancers. This does not mean removing fat from the diet all together. Fat has an essential role in metabolism, in transporting fat soluble vitamins, and as part of our neural cellular structure. The key is the type and amount of fat.

Unsaturated fats are preferable to saturated fats, because saturated fats will be deposited along the walls of the arteries by low density lipoproteins (LDLs). This results in a condition called atherosclerosis which gives rise to high blood pressure and heart problems. Of interest high density lipoproteins (HDLs) carry saturated fats away from the arteries. Exercise and foods such as onions, garlic and nuts stimulate the production of HDLs.

We need to be keenly aware of the sources of saturated fat in our diet. If fat comes from an animal with a liver or if it comes from a source that sounds tropical such as coconut oil, coconut milk, and chocolate then it is saturated. So to limit our intake of saturated fats we simply need to keep the animal protein we eat to a minimum and avoid commercially baked products. However, the most effective method of limiting fat intake to the recommended 25-30% of calories is to use the added fats very sparingly. That is creams, sauces, high fat dairy items, gravies, oils, margarine and butter. We should allow our bodies to obtain the fat it needs in protein and to do this without guilt.

Water

Water is an essential nutrient, as it comprises approximately 55% of our total body weight and 70% of muscle tissue. Water plays a vital role in maintaining our blood volume and therefore the transportation of nutrients and wastes from the cells through the blood. As a natural coolant it helps to regulate the body's temperature. Water is also a medium for energy production and fat oxidation. Inadequate consumption of water may result in feelings of lethargy and fatigue as well as muscle cramping and headaches. The recommended water intake is 30-50 ml. per kilogram of body weight or for the average individual 8 glasses of water per day.

Micronutrients

A balanced diet provides more than 50 important nutrients daily. Inadequate intakes of food cannot be compensated with vitamin / mineral supplements. Multivitamins may contain a fraction of the available micronutrients and none of the macronutrients (carbohydrates, proteins and fats) which provide essential energy to the body. Nor do they provide fiber. For many people vitamins may provide a psychological benefit and using vitamins is not harmful, providing the vitamins and minerals are supplemented in recommended amounts.

There are some instances where supplements are needed:

■ Vitamin D & Calcium for individuals who do not consume foods from the Milk and Milk Products group.

CHAPTER 5

- Vitamin D for individuals who do not include milk in their food intake but who do eat cheese and yogurt.

- Iron & Folacin for pregnant and lactating (breast-feeding) women.

- Vitamin B_{12} for vegetarians who consume few if any foods from animal origin.

- Vitamin B_6 for women using oral contraceptives and to alleviate symptoms of premenstrual syndrome (PMS).

- Fluoride for children over 6 months whose drinking water does not contain fluoride.

Calcium is an important nutrient. It provides strength and structure to the bones and teeth and is necessary for blood clotting and transmitting signals throughout the nervous system. Calcium also plays a role in the function of muscular and hormonal systems. Milk, yogurt, ice cream, cheese, vegetables (particularly green vegetables such as broccoli and spinach), and fish all contain calcium. Due to demands on the female body, girls and women must be particularly diligent about their calcium intake. Teenage girls require the same amount of calcium found in 2 1/2 to 3 1/2 glasses of milk per day (800 to 1000 milligrams or 2 1/2 to 3 1/2 ounces of calcium) and women need the equivalent of 2 1/3 glasses of milk per day (700 milligrams or

almost 2 1/2 ounces of calcium). Because of the threat of osteo-porosis, some experts have proposed that women should be receiving 1000 to 1500 milligrams (3 1/2 to 5 ounces) of calcium per day, or the equivalent of 3 to 4 cups of milk. For individuals allergic to dairy products or who simply do not like them, calcium supplements may be an alternative. Prior to embarking on this course of action a trained and knowledge-able dietician should be consulted.

Make sure your diet contains an adequate source of iron. Iron plays a key role in keeping energy levels up, because it helps the blood transport oxygen from the lungs to the rest of the body. Iron is not produced by the body; it must be ingested. Dietary sources of iron include: dark green vegetables; fruits, such as bananas, apricots, and blueberries; seeds, such as sunflower and sesame seeds; whole grains; eggs; red meat; and poultry. Although organ meats, such as kidney and liver, are high in iron, these organs filter and metabolize preservatives and toxins. Some of these substances are retained in the organs. Therefore, if too much is eaten, these same preservatives and toxins are ingested. Liver is also high in cholesterol.

Avoid the unnecessary use of antacids which may cause depletion of phosphorous and accompanying calcium stores, thus weakening the bones. Some

YOUNG AS YOU LOOK

antacids have been promoted as calcium supplements. A balanced diet of calcium-rich food or the proper use of calcium supplements is preferable to the use of antacids.

Vitamins A, C, and E (antioxidants) help to quench age-promoting chemicals (oxygen-free radicals) released by the body. Many scientists believe these free radicals, which cause a reaction known as oxidization, to be among the major factors in aging. It is thought that damage to cells and molecules can be prevented by the ingestion of vitamin antioxidants which act like a S.W.A.T. team isolating terrorists. Supplements may be useful in reasonable but not excessive doses, although this is controversial. Excessive doses of vitamin A may cause bone pain, hair loss, and dry skin. Vitamin C in excess may precipitate kidney stones. The usual recommended dosages are: vitamin C - 1 gram per day and vitamin E - 400 international units twice daily. Taking low doses of these vitamins is relatively risk free, yet the benefits may be significant.

Zinc, as well as vitamins A, C, and E, may augment the body's defense, or immune system. The immune system is important for the prevention of skin cancers, the disposal of harmful cellular debris, and the repair of aging cells. The usual recommended dosage of zinc sulphate is 220 milligrams daily. As with vitamins, the "benefit-to-risk" ratio may be high, although zinc sulphate remains a controversial supplement.

When vitamins are ingested in mega-doses they can reach toxic levels and the possible side effects may result in permanent damage to vital organs and in the case of vitamins A and D, death. Some of the potential effects of excessive amounts of vitamins are included in the table on page 76.

Daily Eating Habits

Our bodies are a dynamic energy system with a constant demand for fuel. This is achieved through eating. For optimal energy and long lasting satiety a diet high in fiber and low in fat is recommended.

Our daily eating habits help to meet our optimal energy requirements and our nervous system tells us when this has been accomplished. The hypothalamus in our brains is the control center that tells us when to eat and when to stop. It does this by responding to the level of sugar in our blood and to feedback from the vagus nerve and its network of sensors which surround the stomach and duodenum (first section of the small intestine). The body wants what is good for it and the vagus nerve is the informer which tells central control whether or not you are meeting your bodies nutritional needs. It records the value of the food you eat such as complex

Vitamin	Possible Side Effects of Excessive Amounts
A	Fatigue, malaise, headache, loss of hair, loss of nails, aching bones, cerebral edema, vomiting, skin changes, fever, enlarged liver.
D	High blood calcium levels, kidney damage, growth retardation.
E	Headache, nausea, fatigue, dizziness, blurred vision, changes in epithelial tissue.
K	Irritation of the skin and respiratory tract.
C	Nausea, diarrhea, excessive absorbtion of iron (especially in men), kidney stones, rebound scurvy in infants born to women who took high doses of vitamin C during pregnancy.
Niacin	Flushing, itching, persistent skin changes, tachycardia (rapid heart beat), liver damage, high blood sugar, high blood uric acid which may present as gout.
Pyroxidine	Liver disease.
Folate	May antagonize protective effect of dilantin in people with epilepsy.

carbohydrates and proteins as well as the form of the food you eat, for example an apple versus apple juice. There is no getting away from it, our bodies know best and we cannot trick them through mind games. A commitment to eating well will result in our bodies serving us well.

There are certain bad habits to avoid:

■ Skipping meals, especially breakfast immediately sends the body into a preservation mode, where it starts to break down lean body mass to produce its own glucose. This results in a slowing of our metabolism and a triggered response for the next meal to be stored as fat. This is a definite prescription for weight gain.

■ Snacking continually on simple carbohydrates such as cookies and chips never satisfies the body's need to feel full. Or conversely eating three large meals daily with second helpings to ensure that you are stuffed so you won't be tempted to snack between meals is also not the answer.

Remember the body is a dynamic energy system which requires small frequent bursts of fuel. Current research suggests that highly successful weight management occurs with 3 small, well balanced meals and 2 to 3 nutritious snacks every day. The body needs fuel every 2 to 4 hours and hunger is the physiological mechanism which triggers the need. So tune into your hunger and feel the energy surge when you respond appropriately.

Women and men for decades have fallen prey to the idea that weight loss occurs only with strict adherence to a calorie reduced diet. However, the latest research indicates that weight loss induced by inadequate calories results primarily in losses of water and muscle and only a minimal amount of fat.

Our bodies need a certain amount of calories daily just to meet the needs of our basic organ function. This is referred to as a basal metabolic requirement (BMR). When calorie consumption is low our metabolism is compromised and we adapt to the deprivation by becoming more efficient metabolically, which triggers an increase in the storage of fat. This explains why the diet industry continues to be a 30 billion dollar a year industry and 99% of people who lose weight through calorie restriction regain it back within 5 years.

There are no miracles; there are no quick fixes. Healthy, permanent weight loss will occur when the calories you ingest are not below your basal metabolic requirement (BMR) and are not in excess of your energy needs. Ideal loss of fat occurs slowly and requires a commitment to a lifestyle change.

Consult a Registered Dietitian to carefully plan your energy needs and the appropriate partition of calories, as well as the timing of meals and snacks. The rest depends on your tenacity to stick to it. Individuals spend years working against their bodies to this end. Changing your outlook and lifestyle will not only enhance greater physical energy but will reinforce a positive feeling of being in control. It is totally liberating for a chronic dieter to realize this goal and slowly develop a nurturing attitude towards their body and their well-being.

A Word About Diet Medications

Drugs to suppress the appetite, to speed the metabolism, or even to reduce fat from being absorbed in the intestine are making their way into medicine cabinets. For example, Redux, a pill that suppresses the appetite with amphetamine-like action has commanded hundreds of millions of dollars of sales in America.

Xenical, a drug that inhibits the enzyme lipase which breaks down lipids, is poised to enter the mainstream weight reduction market in North America. Taken with meals it prevents up to 30% of ingested fat from entering the intestine and later the bloodstream. By reducing absorption less fat is available for energy or storage in the body's fat depots.

Are these drugs desirable and safe? In the short term yes, but in the long run we do not know. Many questions remain unanswered:

■ Is our dependence on weight control unhealthy physically and psychologically?

■ Over the years how do these drugs affect fat soluble vitamins and other agents that move with fat into our body?

■ How is our sense of control and self-esteem affected?

■ What happens when we stop taking the drugs?

It is too early to really know. When possible, control of body weight through exercise and natural nutritional means, as well as a healthy dose of self acceptance, is clearly more desirable.

EXERCISE

Exercise is essential to a healthy lifestyle, playing an important role in maintaining required weight, as well as affecting the psyche. It is a key player in the ability to grow old gracefully.

Although exercise does not seem to prolong life, it does slow the decline. Some scientists speculate that the inevitable decrease in biological capacity as you age may be halved if you engage in regular aerobic activity. Others claim that people who exercise consistently may expect to live an additional two years. What remains irrefutable, however, is that exercise enhances the joy of life.

Benefits of Exercise

Exercise affects the way we look and feel, as well as our overall health.

Appearance

As time passes, a person's subcutaneous fat stores tend to increase. Women may find that they begin to add inches to their abdomen, arms, hips and buttocks, while men have a tendency to develop love handles and pot bellies. These changes are not necessarily demonstrated on the scale. A woman may weigh 61 kilograms (135 pounds) when she is 25 and the same at 55. Skin fold caliper measurements of the subcutaneous fat is where the differences are definitively demonstrated. At age 25 the normal percentage of body fat is 25%. At age 55 this measurement increases to 30.5%.

These changes in the way in which fat is stored is associated with the aging process, therefore, a lean, fit body at any age has the appearance of being more youthful. A fit body is a shapely body. The curves are in the right place, so that clothing looks and feels more attractive.

Well Being

There is a scientific link between our sense of well being and exercise. This exercise induced sense of well being is attributed to a psychochemical phenomenon in which morphine-like chemicals known as endorphins and enkephalins are released in the brain. These chemicals improve our mood and help us to feel more energetic. A few minutes of exercise, rather than a snooze on the couch, goes a long way to replenishing our energy stores. An increase of energy results in an increase in productivity which in turn contributes to our sense of enjoyment and our quality of life.

A mind-body awareness is developed with regular exercise which contributes to a greater sense of self. This conscious awareness of ones self leads to a greater respect for our health and a better sense of control over our lives. Self confidence and self-esteem increase. We begin to do things for ourselves, resisting the influence of others, because we are in better tune with our own wants, needs, and desires. In fact, bad habits like smoking and alcohol

consumption, may fade in their addictive power as a result of participating in a regular exercise program.

Psychological tests show that people who exercise are more self confident and optimistic. They also demonstrate fewer aberrant mental symptoms, such as helplessness, anxiety, and withdrawal, and are better equipped to deal with stress. In fact, exercise has been reported to be more effective than psychotherapy or antidepressant drugs in treating mild depression.

Health

When people who are sedentary are compared to people who exercise regularly and are considered to be very fit, the sedentary group are 65% more likely to suffer a heart attack or stroke or to develop cancer or diabetes. Participating in a regular exercise program reduced this risk of getting a serious illness to 10%.

These statistics are a very powerful argument for exercising regularly. However, the role of exercise in maintaining an ideal weight has more general appeal than the scare tactics of future illness, until of course those illnesses raise their ugly heads.

Physiologists agree that a moderate fat increase is inevitable as you grow older. Do not despair however, because they also concur that exercise, combined with a sensible dietary intake, is the most effective method to control this aging phenomenon.

Dieting is not the answer. Ninety percent of people who try to lose weight through dieting alone fail. This is because the body perceives that a war is being waged against it and in all likelihood the body will win. Why? Because the body will respond to the threat of starvation by becoming more efficient at storing fat, which it perceives as being vital to its future survival.

About one-third of the weight lost from all diets is lean tissue, not fat tissue. Dieting trains the body to slow the metabolism so that it does not efficiently break down fatty substances in the diet. So, although you may lose weight while you are on the diet, when you begin to eat normal well balanced meals again, you will not only gain the lost weight but you will find that more pounds are being added. This is known as the yo-yo syndrome where an individual may lose 8 pounds initially, but over a period of time regain 10 pounds (4 to 5 kilograms). The body has become very efficient at storing fat for the next period of starvation hence the regained pounds are primarily fat.

The ideal weight control program includes a nutritionally balanced diet combined with an aerobic exercise program. This is easier to say than to implement. That is because the third compo-

nent of an ideal weight control program is the psychological commitment to change. The odds are against you if you do not address the fact that your present lifestyle is probably inconsistent with your desire to control your weight. You must be prepared to make an emotional commitment to change your lifestyle or you will fail to meet your goal of obtaining the ideal weight and level of fitness for your particular body type.

Exercise alone is more effective than diet alone for fat reduction particularly when crash dieting is used rather than slow, progressive change in eating habits.

The Most Effective Exercise

Prolonged endurance activities, such as brisk walking, jogging, cycling or cross-country skiing, are particularly effective in mobilizing fat stores. Because these activities are weight bearing they also play an important role in the prevention of osteoporosis, a disease in which the bones are deplete of calcium. The leanest athletes are runners and weight trainers. Swimmers tend to have a higher percentage of body fat than other similarly-trained athletes. Aerobic exercise not only promotes weight loss, but also helps in maintaining ideal weight.

The reason aerobic exercise is so beneficial is that it enhances the muscle tissue and trains the body to

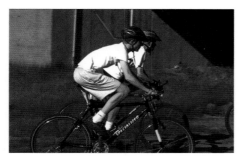

draw on its stores of fat for energy. After about 20 minutes of endurance exercise, the body shifts from primarily using carbohydrates to burning up proportionally more fat.

Weight training has become popular in recent years. One concern that many women, in particular, have is that lifting weights will turn them into female versions of Arnold Schwarzenegger. It is unlikely that women will develop exceptionally large muscles unless they take hormonal supplements. Men, on the other hand, will develop a muscular physique through weight training because they have the requisite testosterone levels to create this effect.

The advantage of weight training is that a finely tuned muscle is more efficient at using the fuel the body receives through food. It also sculpts the body into a more youthful physique.

Some women find that their abdomen and buttocks remain fat despite their participation in regular aerobic exercise and weight training programs. Scientists have found an enzyme, called lipoprotein lipase, that acts to mobilize fat stores in our bodies. For some unknown reason, the activity of this enzyme is compromised in post-menopausal women, particularly in the abdominal and buttock regions. Therefore, it becomes more difficult to get rid of fat in these areas. This is why liposuction has proven to be so popular. Once fat is removed and a constant weight and fitness level are maintained, it is unlikely to return.

How Much Exercise?

It is necessary to exercise aerobically for at least a half-hour 4 times a week in order to effect a substantial change in your body. An aerobic exercise program should begin gradually, as little as 10 minutes at the onset of the program, especially for those individuals who have a sedentary lifestyle. To prepare the body both psychologically and physiologically, approximately 10 to 15 minutes should be spent warming up prior to the aerobic portion of the program and another 10 to 15 minutes cooling down after the more intense middle portion. Warm-up exercises could simply be slower paced walking or cycling. Calisthenic exercises may be included in the cool-down portion.

Regular exercise increases the metabolic rate for up to 24 hours after a workout.

CHAPTER 5

The intensity of the exercise is also important. Moderate exercise appears to be more effective in mobilizing fat stores than highly intensive exercise.

To determine a moderate action pulse rate, subtract your age from 220 and multiply this figure by 70% (.70). Fat utilization by the body is maximized at this pulse rate. Fat burn-off falls precipitously at 80 to 90% of an individual's theoretical pulse rate.

Myths About Exercise

You cannot rid yourself of body fat by "sweating" it off. Ultimately, with extremely rigorous exercise, you can create the equivalent of 3 quarts of fluid per hour. After you replace this fluid, however, you will simply be replacing these lost pounds.

There is also no such thing as spot reducing. Fat gain and distribution tend to be inherited and when weight is lost, body fat is lost proportionally all over. Bouncing on the floor or rolling the hips won't use those stores: a major blow to the popularity of calisthenics. Waistline twists, bends, and leg kicks to reduce thigh size have been supplanted by aerobic exercise. During aerobic exercise fat stores are mobilized from all over the body, including the abdomen and buttocks.

Some people worry that if exercise is stopped muscles will be

converted into fat. It is simply not possible for muscle to be transformed into fat or fat into muscle. They are two separate types of tissues. Muscle loses its bulk due to lack of use or disease. Muscle fiber size is enhanced through exercise particularly weight training. Fat accumulates if the exercise program is discontinued and caloric intake is maintained or increased.

There is no quick and easy way to lose weight or get into shape. Devices such as sauna suits and vibrating machines are not effective and, in addition, can be harmful.

Motivating Yourself to Exercise

A fitness evaluation is, in itself, motivating. Visit an exercise physiologist or a certified fitness appraiser who will determine your cardiorespiratory fitness level, lung function, percentage of body fat, muscle strength, and flexibility. You will also be consulted about the

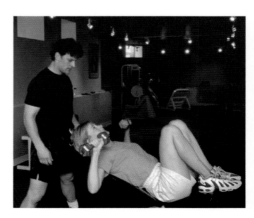

type, frequency, and intensity of exercise you wish to engage in, depending upon the goals you aim to achieve. Keep in mind that there is a distinction between a fitness expert and a fitness enthusiast. Many actors and actresses are in reality fitness enthusiasts. They do a good job of selling fitness. Their books often are more "pep" talk than substance. This does not necessarily preclude a fitness enthusiast from also being an expert, but this is the exception rather than the rule. Be cautious! Often a book may tend to focus on only one aspect of physical fitness, for example, flexibility.

Exercise with a friend or in a group. Join a fitness club. You have to be very self-motivated to exercise consistently by yourself. If you do wish to exercise alone, however, be sure to purchase good quality equipment.

Keep an exercise diary, noting the type of activity, your pulse rate, the distance cycled, and so forth. Some individuals also keep a concurrent food diary.

If you are 35 or older, and are not accustomed to vigorous activity, consult your family practitioner prior to beginning an exercise program.

CHAPTER 5

PART

II

Medical Alternatives:
Enhancing Your Appearance

The *Face & Neck*

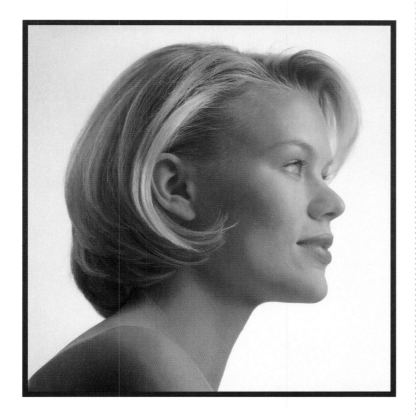

In spite of the natural care you give to the skin on your face and neck, sometimes nature needs a helping hand. Fortunately, you live in an age when medical knowledge has advanced to where it can help you look your best at any age.

CHAPTER 6

Various medications and surgical techniques have been developed specifically to correct nature's missteps, and to reverse the effects that aging has had upon your face and neck.

O*ur agenda for a youthful face and neck includes:*

■ *medicated creams*
■ *injections for reducing wrinkles*

Where had the time gone? Sandra was approaching her 50th birthday. Her youngest son had left home and her first grandchild had been born. Yet she did not feel old or grandmotherly. Her work as a marketing consultant was satisfying and she loved the freedom from the demands and worries of motherhood. Her divorce had not been easy and she hoped that some day she would be able to form a bond with someone new. Yet, in the back of her mind was the nagging doubt about her age and how she looked.

Sandra knew she looked her age, if not older. Her skin had the ruddy complexion that comes with too much sun exposure: fine blood vessels covered her nose and cheeks and the texture and color of her skin was uneven. Worry lines had etched their way into her forehead and around her lips. In fact, people frequently commented on how concerned she looked.

It was the day she was listening to a dermatologist speaking on the radio about what could be done to reduce the signs of aging that she realized it was her turn. Several months later, after the regular use of medicated creams, laser resurfacing to smooth out the texture, color and wrinkles on her

face, as well as vascular laser therapy for her blood vessels a friend asked her what she had done to look so good.

Sandra's case demonstrates that the way you look affects the way others perceive you. The head and neck are the most visible body parts: they are what people notice first. Based on their first impressions of your face, hair, and neck they will draw conclusions about the state of your health, emotions, age, and beauty.

The face and neck provide the first clues to age, through pigment and texture changes, wrinkles, and sagging skin. A closer look at the current therapeutic options available to lessen these signs of aging will demonstrate that you do not have to play the cards nature has dealt.

The previous section on the skin discussed what you can do to maintain the skin on your face without medical intervention. In this section, the medical options for restoration of the skin are reviewed, showing you how advances in medical technology make it possible for you to look your best.

A number of medical options are currently available for the removal or reduction of wrinkles. Some involve regular application of a medicated cream or lotion to the face (topical agents), while other methods require surgical procedures.

CHAPTER 6

MEDICATED CREAMS

Medicated creams containing tretinoin and alpha hydroxy acids have captured and held the attention of the media for nearly a decade. Yet neither of these ingredients are new to dermatologists, who have been prescribing their use in the management of skin diseases such as acne, eczema, and psoriasis for years. It is the use of these agents to combat aging that has attracted so much attention.

Tretinoin

Tretinoin is the chemical name for one member of a family of compounds called retinoids, which are related to vitamin A. Vitamin A acts at the cellular level to encourage both the secretion of mucus between the cells and normal cell development. It is uncertain how tretinoin specifically affects the biological function of skin cells, although it is thought to thin the top layer of the skin and to increase its blood supply. This accelerates the rate at which the skin is renewed. Tretinoin is also thought to improve the alignment of collagen in the dermis, preventing it from clumping up, as occurs with sun-related wrinkling.

Much of the initial improvement seen with tretinoin is likely caused by the swelling of skin due to irritation. Fluid shifts occur with inflammation, and this temporarily smoothes out the fine wrinkles. Subsequently, the collagen realigns itself and a more permanent reversal of wrinkling occurs.

Research has shown two additional benefits of tretinoin. It has proven effective in reducing or eliminating precancerous, sun damaged spots. It also changes the

---

THE BENEFITS OF TRETINOIN

1. Fluid shifts due to moderate inflammation puff up the skin causing fine wrinkles to become less obvious.

2. Long-term use alters various structures in the skin making it more youthful (rosy, soft, less wrinkled).

3. Pigment spots become lighter and the over-all color of the skin evens out.

4. Precancerous scaly spots often disappear.

5. Blackheads surface and slough because the dead lining around the pores peels.

6. Pus-filled pimples dry up.

skin's ability to retain water by increasing its mucus levels. By raising the water content of the skin, wrinkles swell and become less obvious.

Tretinoin is available by prescription in products such as Stieva-A, Retisol-A, Vitamin A Acid, Retin-A, Rejuva-A, and Renova. It is the variation in concentrations and vehicles in which the tretinoin are carried that differentiate between these products. For example Stieva-A and Retin-A are carried in gels, creams, and liquids in concentrations which vary from 0.01% (low) to 0.1% (high).

Retisol-A is carried in a moisturizing cream which also contains a PABA-free broad spectrum sunscreen which protects against UVA and UVB rays of light. The moisturizing base is non-comedogenic so it does not aggravate acne-prone skin. It can be obtained in concentrations varying from 0.01% to 0.1%. For the busy individual who does not want to fuss with a lot of different creams this is an excellent option.

Rejuva-A and Renova contain mid-level concentrations of tretinoin. Like Retisol-A these products marry the benefits of

Tretinoin

Trade Name	Company	Vehicle	
Retin-A	Ortho-McNeil	Gel:	0.01%, 0.025%
		Cream:	0.01%, 0.025%, 0.05%, 0.1%
Renova	Ortho-McNeil	Cream:	0.05%
Stieva-A	Stiefel	Gel:	0.01%, 0.025%, 0.05%
		Cream:	0.01%, 0.025%, 0.05%, 0.1%
		Liquid:	0.025%, 0.05%
Rejuva	Stiefel	Cream:	0.025%
Retisol-A	Stiefel	Cream:	0.01%, 0.025%, 0.05%, 0.1%
Vitamin A Acid	Rorer	Gel:	0.01%, 0.025%, 0.05%
		Cream:	0.01%, 0.025%, 0.05%, 0.1%

Y O U N G   A S   Y O U   L O O K

tretinoin and noncomedogenic moisturizers. The goal is to control the redness and irritation that is problematic with higher concentrations of tretinoin.

Will tretinoin reduce all the signs of aging?

Tretinoin is not a magical elixir of youth. It is most useful for reducing fine wrinkles in areas which are noticeably sun damaged for example, around the eyes, nose, and mouth, especially in fair skinned individuals. It is also effective for harmonizing skin texture and color. Tretinoin has little or no effect on sagging skin or deep furrows, but the use of tretinoin in combination with other techniques, such as laser resurfacing or surgical implants, can noticeably improve the skin.

The more extensive the damage to the skin from age and environmental assaults, the more aggressive the treatment must be. Laser resurfacing, liposuction and surgical lifts are alternatives which need to be considered as the changes to the skin become more involved.

Claims have been made that tretinoin may actually prevent wrinkles. From the time sun damage occurs, 5 to 20 years may go by before the skin exhibits any signs of injury. The use of tretinoin at an early age, therefore, may or may not have a long-term effect in preventing wrinkles from occurring. This remains an area of

controversy. Sunscreens, however, are a proven form of protection.

How should tretinoin be applied?

Tretinoin is available in creams of various concentrations. Since higher concentrations may irritate the skin, it is wise to start off with a weaker preparation and build up to a stronger one. This is especially important to people with dry or sensitive skin. Those with less sensitive skin can begin with a higher concentration. Close-up photographs are a useful way of monitoring improvement with tretinoin, as it is difficult to note any on a daily basis.

The following steps are recommended for using tretinoin:

■ Wash the face with a mild soap, dry gently, and wait about 20 minutes for the skin to replenish its natural oils.

■ Apply tretinoin to the entire face with approximately three dabs: one for the forehead, one for the area around the eyes and across the nose, and one around the mouth and lower face. Using more will not accelerate its effectiveness. It may, instead, cause irritation, and treatment with tretinoin would have to be stopped until the skin has recovered. Those with sensitive or dry skin should avoid the delicate skin around the eyes and mouth when first using tretinoin or use a milder concentration in these areas, then gradually build up the strength which is used.

■ If the skin shows signs of dryness, apply a moisturizer after applying the tretinoin.

■ Use a sunscreen with an SPF of at least 15. Sunscreens should be reapplied throughout the day according to the amount of time spent in the sun. As mentioned, Retisol-A combines both a moisturizer and a broad spectrum sunscreen with the tretinoin.

■ Avoid using astringents or toners since they contain drying agents, such as citrus fruits (lemon and lime) or alcohol. These agents aggravate skin dryness and irritation.

Progress should be monitored by a dermatologist who will increase the concentration as discomfort and irritation disappear. If irritation is excessive, see a dermatologist immediately.

After a year of daily tretinoin use, the number of applications may be reduced while maintaining the same effect. For best results, however, a maintenance program should be adopted in consultation with a dermatologist.

We have found that 19 out of 20 people can tolerate tretinoin and are happy with the results within six months, provided they are able to use a concentration of 0.05% or higher on a daily basis.

Is tretinoin safe?

Tretinoin is safe. It has also been approved by the FDA in the United States as an effective means of treating wrinkles. Because it is classified as a drug it must be prescribed and monitored by an informed medical practitioner.

Mild to severe dryness of the skin may occur, especially in the early stages of use. This can be controlled by a gradual increase in concentration or by using moisturizers in conjunction with higher doses.

Redness and irritation, as well as itching, burning, and tingling sensations have also been reported. These tend to occur when the skin has sloughed off its dry layer and is producing new skin cells. If much discomfort is experienced, the dosage may be reduced and an anti-inflammatory agent, such as a mild cortisone salve, may be applied.

Since tretinoin intensifies the susceptibility to sunburn, sunscreens must be used. In fact, sunscreens should be a part of the daily regimen, as the sun is a major cause of wrinkling and skin cancers.

Although, at this point in time, there is no documented reason why pregnant women should not use tretinoin, it is probably better to be on the safe side and avoid its use until the baby is born.

Alpha Hydroxy Acids

Alpha hydroxy acids (AHA) are becoming a popular alternative to tretinoin in the battle against photo aging because they tend to be less irritating and drying to the skin. They may also be used in conjunction with tretinoin to achieve synergistic benefits

Often referred to as fruit acids because they are found in plants and foods such as citrus fruits, apples, grapes, sugar cane and sour milk, AHA's have been used to beautify the skin for years. Cleopatra and Marie Antoinette bathed in milk and the upper crust of England softened their skin with red wine.

By breaking down the intra-cellular bonds of the epidermis AHA's accelerate the sloughing of the superficial dead skin cells and thin the outer layer of the skin. Lactic acid and glycolic acid are two AHA's commonly found in dermatologic preparations.

The concentration of the AHA, the base in which it is transmitted to the skin, and the type of AHA all contribute to how effective a product will be.

In low to medium concentrations (4 to 8%) AHA's are used to improve the appearance of age spots, treat acne and clogged pores, and eliminate warts.

In higher concentrations (8 to 12%) they have been found to reduce fine wrinkles and even out irregular skin coloring. A combination of glycolic acid with bleaching agents such as hydroquinone or kojic acid has proven effective in the treatment of age spots and melasma (the mask of pregnancy).

The vehicle in which AHA's are carried can alter the effectiveness of the concentration. If the base buffers the AHA to control for irritation then a 12% concentration may only be as effective as a 5% unbuffered preparation.

The type of alpha hydroxy acid is also of importance in determin-

Age Spots: Treated with Bleaching Creams

BEFORE

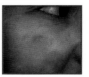

AFTER

PHOTOS
COURTESY OF
DR. DON GROOT

THE BENEFITS OF ALPHA HYDROXY ACIDS

1. Rapid, deep exfoliation of dead skin cells on the surface of the epidermis.

2. Removes debris from clogged pores to assist in the treatment of acne.

3. Reduces fine wrinkles.

4. Evens out irregular skin coloring.

5. With hydroquinone or kojic acid, it lightens age spots and other pigment changes in the skin such as melasma.

CHAPTER 6

ing how effective the product will be. Glycolic acid consists of smaller molecules and therefore penetrates deeper into the epidermis. In high concentrations it may stimulate realignment of the collagen in the dermis.

Lactic acids have a larger molecular structure so they do not penetrate as deeply. However, lactic acids are very effective as chemically enhanced moisturizers. When applied to slightly moist skin products like Lachydrin and Lacticare lotions aid in water retention.

Short of being a biochemist, how do you tell which product is best for you? The first step would be to consult a dermatologist, then it may be a matter of trial and error until you find the product which best suits your skin type.

How should AHA's be applied?

AHA's are applied in a similar fashion to tretinoin:

- Cleanse the face and/or body and wait about 20 minutes so the skin is completely dry and has replenished its natural oils.

- If the AHA you have selected is in a moisturizing base, simply apply the cream. If it is in a nonmoisturizing base, apply the AHA prior to using a moisturizer. If it is applied after the moisturizer it will not penetrate the skin.

- Be sure to use a broad spectrum

sunscreen with an SPF of at least 15.

- Avoid using astringents or toners as they will contribute to dryness and irritation.

The benefits of AHA should be seen within 1 to 4 months, but don't expect miracles. More aggressive treatments are required for deep creases and loose skin.

Are AHA's safe?

Yes AHA's in concentrations of 12% or less are safe and effective. However it is important to understand that skin care products containing AHA's are not simply moisturizers, they may actually affect the structure and function of the skin. It is for this reason that some would argue that AHA's should be classified as drugs and only be made available through a prescription from a doctor.

If dryness and irritation do occur cut back the concentration of the AHA product or reduce the number of applications.

Concentrations greater than 13% could present problems if they are not monitored by a dermatologist. This is where concerns begin to arise with alpha hydroxy peels offered by estheticians. In some cases they are using peeling agents with a concentration of 30% or more. At these levels they are moving into the realm of a controlled chemical burn rather than an aggressive exfoliating

Alpha Hydroxy Acid Products

Product	Acid	Percentage
Alpha Hydrox Face Cream	Glycolic	3%
Avon Anew Perfecting Complex	Glycolic	2-4%
Benefit Glycol 7%	Glycolic	7%
Chanel Formulae Intensive Day Lift Refining Complex	Lactic	not disclosed
Clinique Turnaround Cream	Salicylic	1%
Elizabeth Arden Ceramide	Hydroxy Caprylic	not disclosed
Time Complex Moisture Cream	Synthetic AHA	
Estée Lauder Fruition Triple ReActivating Complex	Glycolic	1.2%
Eucerin Plus Moisturizing Lotion	Lactic	4.1%
Guertain Issima Aquaserum	Lactic	not disclosed
La Prairie Age Management Serum	Lactic	5%
Mary Kay Skin Revival Serum/Cream	Lactic Salicylic	not disclosed
Origins Starting Over	Glycolic Lactic	not disclosed
Pond's Dramatic Results Capsules with Nutrium	Hydroxy caprylic	not disclosed
Prescriptives All You Need	Lactic Tartaric Citric	not disclosed
* LacHydrin 12%	Lactic	12%
* NeoStrata AHA Skin Smoothing Cream	Glycolic	8%
* NeoStrata AHA Sensitive Skin Formula	Glycolic	4%
* Reversa AHA Solution for Oily and Acne Prone Skin	Glycolic	8%
* Reversa AHA Skin Smoothing Cream	Glycolic	8%
* Reversa AHA Skin Smoothing Lotion	Glycolic	10%
* NeoStrata HQ	Glycolic Hydroquinone	10% 2%
* Reversa HQ	Glycolic Hydroquinone	10% 2%

* DENOTES DERMATOLOGIST RECOMMENDED

agent. As there are no standards for training for estheticians and in many instances no medical monitoring we strongly advise that the consumer beware.

Do not use products which have been sitting around and open for a long time. The pH balance may become altered and could severely irritate or even burn the skin.

A Synergistic Approach

Many dermatologists have found that combining the use of tretinoin and glycolic acid with a bleaching agent provides an additive benefit. The regime we recommend to patients is as follows:

■ Cleanse the face in the morning with a mild soap, let dry for 20 minutes and apply Retisol-A in a concentration that suits you. You will recall from our discussion on tretinoin that Retisol-A contains tretinoin, moisturizing agents and a broad spectrum sunscreen with an SPF of 15.

■ In the evening cleanse the face again and wait 20 minutes. Apply a cream, gel or lotion that contains glycolic acid and hydroquinone or kojic acid. The hydroquinone once exposed to the air will turn the product a rusty red. Other than looking a bit unusual this is of no consequence. Kojic acid is just as effective for bleaching discolorations of the skin but does not oxidize when exposed to the air. NeoStrata HQ contains glycolic acid and hydroquinone and Reversa HQ is in a hydro-alcoholic gel base with glycolic acid 10% and hydroquinone 2%.

Antioxidants

You will recall from our discussion in Chapter 5 that oxygen free radicals are thought to be a major player in the aging process. Antioxidants (Vitamins A, C and E) are thought to prevent the formation of these unstable chemicals which damage the cells through a process called oxidation. Scientists have suggested for a number of years that ingestion of antioxidants on a regular basis may help to slow the overall effect of aging on the body.

It was only a matter of time before cosmetic and pharmaceutical companies picked up on the notion of applying antioxidants topically to the skin. As with alpha hydroxy acids, the issue is how much is enough to make a difference and cosmetic preparations usually do not contain high enough concentrations.

It is believed that oxygen free radicals are released when the skin is exposed to the sun and are largely responsible for the photodamage of the lipids, melanin, collagen, and elastins in the skin. Research suggests that topical antioxidants help to prevent the deterioration of the skin over time

YOUNG AS YOU LOOK

by neutralizing these free radicals. Although antioxidants are not a substitute for a broad based sunscreen, they provide protection which is comparable to an SPF of 3.

Stimulation of the production of collagen in the second layer of the skin has also been attributed to antioxidants. Delivery however is the issue. Fat soluble vitamin E penetrates the epidermis with relative ease, however, other vitamin molecules like Vitamin C are too large. They require some type of vehicle for transport to the dermis. Liposomes, tiny fat capsules, are one such vehicle.

Antioxidants have not yet stood the test time, therefore, it is difficult to say for sure whether they actually prevent or repair photo aging of the skin. However, there is probably no harm in trying them as long as the skin is also well protected from the sun. Look for a concentration of at least 10.

SOFT TISSUE IMPLANTS AND INJECTIONS

The use of a topical agent, such as tretinoin, or AHA's, for reduction of fine wrinkles is the simplest intervention option. The process is easy and painless, the potential side effects are not severe, and the cost is reasonable. There are limits, however, to their effectiveness. Other more invasive options exist to reverse the signs of aging which include injections (wrinkle-implant therapy and muscle relaxants), resurfacing techniques (lasabrasions and chemical peels), and surgery (face, eyelid, and brow lifts).

Implant Therapy

Wrinkle implants can best be described as fillers. Substances such as collagen (in its various forms), tissue glue (Hylaform viscoelastic gel), Gore-Tex, SoftForm, fat, or silicone are used to fill furrows, creases, and folds in the skin. These wrinkles are generally deeper than the fine wrinkles caused by sun damage and are often found in areas of muscle pull, for example on either side of the mouth and nose, between the brows, and on the forehead. With the exception of silicone, SoftForm and Gore-Tex, which have unique properties and problems, these agents are organic substances injected into the skin to supplement the facial structures altered with age.

Implants are not new. They were used as early as the nineteenth century. At that time the substances were largely inorganic and included wax, aluminum, gold, cork, ivory, and porcelain. Unfortunately, infections and allergic reactions were common. A classic example was the beautiful Duchess of Marlborough who was once the belle of London society. She became a recluse after a series of liquid paraffin injections caused

Collagen Implant: Wrinkles

BEFORE

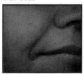

AFTER

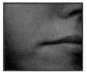

PHOTOS COURTESY OF DR. DON GROOT

ORGANIC IMPLANTS

Advantages:

1. Low-risk procedure.

2. Minimal post-treatment cosmetic disability.

3. Quick fix, lunch time procedure.

4. Subtle to dramatic cosmetic improvement depending on the amount injected.

5. If an allergic reaction occurs, it disappears quickly.

6. Costs less on a per session basis than cosmetic surgery.

Disadvantages:

1. Possibility of allergic reactions even if the test sites are negative.

2. Not a permanent solution; enhancements are required.

3. Ongoing costs with each injection.

4. Precludes individuals with allergies to agents in the implant or who have rheumatoid arthritis.

irreversible allergic reactions which destroyed her beauty. Today, people are more fortunate than the Duchess because the use of soft tissue implants made from organic substances has proven to be highly successful.

What types of implants are available?

Organic implants are made of the following substances: Zyderm and Zyplast collagen suspensions, Koken atelocollagen solution, Fibrel gelatin matrix implant, Hylaform viscoelastic gel and fat (microlipid transfer). Inorganic implants are made of silicone fluid, Gore-Tex or SoftForm. Each differs one from another, and each has both positive and negative attributes.

Collagen is one of the building blocks of skin. Some of the organic implants are forms of collagen which have different agents within their suspensions and solutions. Zyderm, Zyplast, and Koken are bovine collagen. Zyderm and Zyplast originate from the skin of cattle and are milky in appearance, whereas Koken is a clear solution originating from the skin of calves.

A significant breakthrough in soft tissue implants is Hylaform viscoelastic gel. This gel is a derivative of a ubiquitous molecule made of linked starches (polysac-

INORGANIC IMPLANTS

Advantages:

1. Permanent, no touch ups are necessary.

2. Allergic reactions are rare.

Disadvantage:

1. Requires a highly skilled surgeon to avoid misplacement.

2. The implants may migrate out of place.

3. The body may reject the implant through an immune response.

charides) from modified hyaluronan which is located between the structural cells of the skin. It acts as a type of inter-cellular glue.

Fibrel and microlipid transfers both use substances from the patient's own body. Fibrel is unique in that it is composed of gelatin powder and another chemical agent which is mixed with the yellow protein of the recipient's blood.

In the microlipid transfer, fat is taken from one area of the body, usually from underneath the navel, and injected into the furrows or wrinkles of the same person.

Silicone fluid is an artificial solution of silicon, oxygen, and other elements. The use of silicone for injecting into wrinkles has not been approved by the Food and Drug Administration in the United States nor the Health Protection Branch in Canada. Even so, it has been used by numerous practitioners

because of its permanent nature, although it has been less popular since the advent of organic implants.

Medical Gore-Tex has been used to patch blood vessels since the 1970's and in the hands of a skilled practitioner can be effective in the treatment of deep furrows and scars. If it is not properly implanted it can shift out of place. However it is not as unforgiving as silicone as it can be removed if it begins to migrate.

SoftForm facial implants is a new type of sub-dermal (under the skin) implant which is valuable in the treatment of persistent deep furrows. Repeat treatments are not required. The SoftForm facial implant is composed of expanded polytetrafluoroethylene and comes in the shape of a tube. Like Gore-Tex it has a safety record in other areas of medicine. It has been used in over 2 million patients in vascular repair procedures. The purported benefit over Gore-Tex is

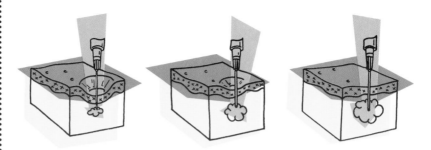

that it is easier to implant, it does not slip out of place, and it is readily removed, if desired. As it is very new in the marketplace, only time will tell whether this is truly the case.

What is involved in implant therapy?

Test sites are important to the success of some implants, including Zyderm, Zyplast, Koken and Fibrel because they minimize the risk of an allergic reaction. Most physicians perform two tests at approximately one month intervals. A small amount of the implant material is injected into the second layer of the skin on the inside of the arm. If the skin becomes inflamed and itchy at the test site then an allergic reaction has occurred. In this case, another type of implant material may be tried. If this is also unsuccessful then implant therapy as an option for the treatment of deep wrinkles

may have to be abandoned.

Although Hylaform viscoelastic gel is in its infant stage as a soft tissue implant, it would appear from all reports that it does not require test sites as allergic reactions are very rare. Microlipid transfers do not require pre-implant tests, because the implant consists of fat from another area of the same body.

Once it has been determined that an allergic reaction will not occur the physician can proceed with the implant therapy. The selected material is injected into the second layer of the skin along the wrinkle. Depending on how deep the crease is, a second layer of implant solution may be required.

If Zyderm or Zyplast are used, the physician will overcorrect, raising the line of the crease above the surface of the skin. This compensates for the anesthetic within the implant solution and will flatten out within a short period of time as the local anesthesia wears off.

Once the implant is in place the physician may massage the treated area to feather out the line of correction.

Gore-Tex and SoftForm implants are not injected but threaded along the furrow or depression targeted for correction. A local anesthetic is used to numb the area before and tiny incisions are made at either end of the insertion line. A tunnel is then created through which the Gore-Tex or SoftForm implant is threaded.

What does the injection site look like afterwards?

Slight blotchiness and swelling is usually evident after the injection of an implant. The degree of swelling varies with the type of implant used. Needle-prick sites and bruising may also be apparent. All evidence of the procedure has usually disappeared within 3 hours to 3 days, except that the furrows and wrinkles are less obvious. In rare instances a bruise may last up to 9 days. Patients who can tolerate the implants without an allergic reaction are generally happy with the results.

Gore-Tex and SoftForm implants require a stitch at either end of the implant site. Once these are removed there is no

visible sign that an implant has been put in place.

Does it hurt to have soft tissue implants?

Some mild discomfort will be experienced, or, at most, moderate pain on the injection of the implant. Zyderm and Zyplast have a local anesthetic in their suspensions and this decreases some of the discomfort. Koken and Fibrel are available with or without anesthetic. Hylaform viscoelastic gel, micro-lipid transfer, and silicone fluid do not have anesthetics in their suspensions and, therefore, tend to be more uncomfortable.

Gore-Tex and SoftForm require local anesthesia at the treatment site prior to the placement of the implant.

How safe are organic implants?

The common organic implants have proven to be relatively safe non-surgical options for the treatment of many skin contour problems, such as wrinkles and furrows.

Hylaform viscoelastic gel is a relatively new implant material so it does not have the track record of such products as Zyderm and Zyplast. However, two decades of investigation would suggest that it will be safe and effective for soft tissue augmentation as it is biologically compatible and stable in dermal tissue. Of interest it also promises to be of importance in other areas of medicine including orthopaedics, ophthalmology, and urology.

The types of problems which may arise from organic implants include:

■ *Allergic reactions:* In 1 to 2% of cases organic implants, with the exception of Hylaform viscoelastic gel implants and microlipid transfers, are regarded by the body as foreign and rejected in an allergic reaction. If there is a history of allergies to the ingredients within the implant solution, or if an allergic reaction occurs at a test site on the arm, implant therapy should not be undertaken. Allergic reactions are characterized by prolonged redness, swelling, itching, and firmness. A reaction usually persists for 3 to 4 months, lasting perhaps a year or longer in more severe cases. On very rare occasions, a scab may form with the subsequent sloughing or shedding of the skin at the treatment site. This may result in a shallow scar.

Delayed allergic reactions may occur even though the test site was found to be normal and one or more implants were successfully injected. For this reason, some physicians repeat the test within a month. If no allergic reaction occurs after the second test, the implants are then injected into the areas requiring treatment.

If a reaction is caused by one type of implant, it is possible another could be used once all signs indicate the previous implant has been absorbed. For example, Zyderm and Zyplast contains a local anesthetic, whereas matrix implants do not. Although a local anesthetic is in most cases beneficial, those allergic to it may wish to try the Koken or Fibrel implants.

■ *Other types of problems:* There is the unlikely chance (less than 1%) that a blood vessel may be hit or blocked during an injection. If this occurs a bruise may form at the site or a scab may occur with subsequent sloughing or shedding of the skin. This could result in a shallow scar. Because this is more likely to occur when treating the vertical creases between the eyebrows some dermatologists are now opting to use localized muscle relaxants (Botox botulinum exotoxin). The relaxants, when injected into the muscles above the eyebrow cause a temporary paralysis so an individual can no longer frown. The temporary muscle inactivity reduces the wrinkles.

If collagen is injected into a vein near the eye, visual loss could occur. Only one incident of this happening out of millions of injections has been reported so the risk is extremely low.

YOUNG AS YOU LOOK

At the time of implant therapy it is wise to avoid the use of aspirin or other types of nonsteroidal anti-inflammatory drugs that reduce the clotting of the blood. This will help control bleeding and bruising at the treatment site.

If there is a history of herpes simplex, the trauma caused by the injection of the collagen may stimulate the eruption of a herpes cold sore at the site of the injection.

■ *Relation to connective tissue disease:* There have been some reports that connective tissue diseases such as rheumatoid arthritis, systemic lupus erythematosus, dermato-myositis and polymyositis may be caused by collagen implants because they have occurred in patients who have no history of these diseases but have received collagen injections. After an intense investigation, the Food and Drug Administration in the United States found that "…there is insufficient statistical or biological evidence to support a conclusion that collagen injections cause auto-immune or connective tissue diseases in persons without a history of these diseases." Yet it would seem prudent that patients with collagen related diseases such as rheumatoid arthritis should not be injected with collagen implants until

new data is available to clarify this issue. An alternative is the use of microlipid (or fat) transfers or the new Hylaform viscoelastic gel.

■ *Safety with pregnancy:* Whether or not implants can be safely injected during pregnancy or breast feeding has not been established, so it is better to wait until after the postnatal period before embarking on an implant therapy program.

What about inorganic implants?

Silicone implants are an alternative to organic substances. Their use, however, is controversial. If incorrectly used, silicone has many potential complications, largely because it is unforgiving. Once silicone is in place, it is permanent. This is good, if properly placed. On the other hand, if a low-grade silicone solution or an unnecessarily large amount is used by an unskilled clinician, the error is permanent. This is because silicone is not slowly absorbed by the body as in the case of the organic implants.

Silicone may be perceived by the body as "foreign", and reactions may occur in the form of an allergic granuloma (or bump). Tracking or migration of silicone from one site to another is also a potential problem which results in unsightly bumps away from the

CHAPTER 6

area being treated. If high-grade medical silicone is injected by a skilled physician, using a micro-injection technique, the likelihood of adverse reactions is extremely small. In fact, until recently, silicone implants were undergoing a revival in North America. However, the questionable association with auto-immune disease is still unclear to both researchers and lay people. It is for this reason that there is currently a moratorium on the use of injectable silicone.

Gore-Tex and SoftForm are remarkably stable agents and allergic reactions are virtually unheard of. Never-the-less they are foreign materials and our body's immune system will sometimes wall off foreign matter with a protective fibrous coat or at worst it will try to expel the foreign body. In these rare instances the implant would have to be removed.

How long do implants last?

Organic implants are only temporary solutions and require touch ups from time to time. The body's metabolism slowly reduces the bulk of these fillers or implants. Depending on the area of the body being injected, the rate of metabolism, and the type of implant, the frequency with which touch ups are required varies. Different studies report different findings. Most Zyderm collagen implants require touch ups within

3 to 6 months, and Zyplast collagen implants require them between 6 to 9 months. Occasionally, the implant will be metabolized within a few days or weeks. Our experience has been that consumption of alcohol or exposure to sun and heat increases the rate of metabolism and the subsequent reduction of the injected collagen, as well as an increase in the risk of an allergic reaction.

Studies suggest that on average Koken atelocollagen solution metabolizes within 8 to 14 months, although our experience has been that Koken is metabolized in 3 to 6 months.

Early studies suggest that the Fibrel gelatin-matrix implant may last longer than Zyderm or Zyplast, however, we have found that it lasts no longer than Zyplast, 6 to 9 months. When injected into a pitted scar, approximately 80% of it is still present after one year. Its disappearance and migration is faster in wrinkles because of the additional muscle movement.

The new kid on the block, Hylaform viscoelastic gel, promises to last longer than the other implant materials, but this has yet to be confirmed through regular use and reporting.

The staying power of microlipid transfers (moving fat from one spot to another) is extremely variable depending largely on whether or not the fat "takes", that is, actually develops its own sustaining blood supply in the new site. Some reports suggest that they seem to metabolize much faster than other organic agents, and other reports indicate that they either entirely disappear or remain permanently.

Since the inorganic implants (silicone, Gore-Tex and SoftForm) are not metabolized, no touch ups are required. If they are not properly injected or inserted or if they migrate out of place due to gravity or muscle pull, they will not be absorbed with time and will be permanently displaced. In these instances Gore-Tex and SoftForm can be removed, silicone cannot.

Can the implants be used in other ways?

The signs of aging around the mouth are cosmetically annoying to many women. Collagen is used to add definition to the fading borders of the lips and to soften the fine lines around the mouth. The implant material is injected along the vermilion borders of the upper and lower lips and into any deep furrows extending out from the lip. Women delight in the fact that their lipstick no longer bleeds into the wrinkles around their mouth. However, collagen implants must be repeated to maintain their effectiveness. For a more permanent solution, laser resurfacing should be considered.

Large well defined lips are also

one of today's signatures of beauty and this same technique is used to augment the lips of women of all ages. To add further definition to the heart shaped area of the upper lip, known as the Cupid's Bow, the collagen is injected into the vertical ridges between the upper lip and the nose.

Some cosmetic surgeons may also inject collagen into the red fleshy part of the lips to plump them up. The risk of hitting a small blood vessel exists and if this should happen, crusting and loss of some lip tissue may occur. It is for this reason, except in exceptional circumstances, implants are best limited to the outline of the lip.

How much does it cost and who performs this procedure?

Cost varies with the location, the expertise of the practitioner, and the type and amount of implant used. The average cost for a test site prior to the actual implantation may range from $80 to $120. The range in price to the patient per ampoule of implant may vary from $200 to $500 depending on the type of implant and the amount used. The average patient requires 1 to 4 ampoules per treatment and the number of treatment sessions varies.

Dermatologists, plastic surgeons and other cosmetic surgeons perform all forms of implant surgery. Because the cosmetic result with inorganic implants is so

Collagen Implant: Lips

BEFORE

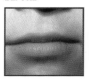

AFTER

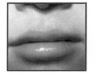

PHOTOS COURTESY OF DR. DON GROOT

operator dependant and even then somewhat risky, many surgeons have mixed feelings about their use. Nurse practitioners under the watchful eye of a surgeon, will in some cases inject certain types of organic soft tissue implants, such as Zyplast and Zyderm.

Muscle Relaxant Injections

Ophthalmologists use an injectable toxin known as Botox (botulinum exotoxin) to prevent muscles from contracting in compulsive eye squinting and to weaken strong eye muscles that induce wandering eyes in children.

This same technique is used to block movement in wrinkle creating muscles. Botox is particularly effective in ironing out the deep creases on the lower forehead between the eye brows. It has also been used to treat the small lines (crow's feet) spreading from the corners of the eyes, forehead wrinkles and neck folds.

What is involved in Botox injections?

The procedure takes only a few minutes and consists of injecting the toxin into the muscle of the offending area. It causes slight discomfort, a sense of burning as the solution enters the muscle. This only lasts for the length of the injection. Within 48 hours, the muscle begins to weaken, and within 7 to 10 days its movement is completely lost. The muscle is not damaged; it is just temporarily immobilized.

How long will the Botox last?

Muscle movement gradually returns over 4 to 6 months, depending on the amount of toxin used. However as the body adjusts to the idea that those muscles are not available for use, the learned behavior of muscle contraction in response to a stimuli is forgotten. Unless the old behaviour is relearned the results may be permanent.

Is Botox safe?

Botox has been used by ophthalmologists since 1980. Side effects are rare and may include a small bruise at the sight of the injection or a slight drooping (ptosis) of the eyelid. The latter occurs in 1% of people and is temporary.

There has never been any reported damage to the eyes.

Who gives Botox injections and how much does it cost?

Dermatologists, ophthalmologists, and other cosmetic surgeons trained in the technique will use Botox injections as one of the many treatment modalities available to combat wrinkles.

CHAPTER 6

The *Face & Neck*

THE WAY YOU LOOK

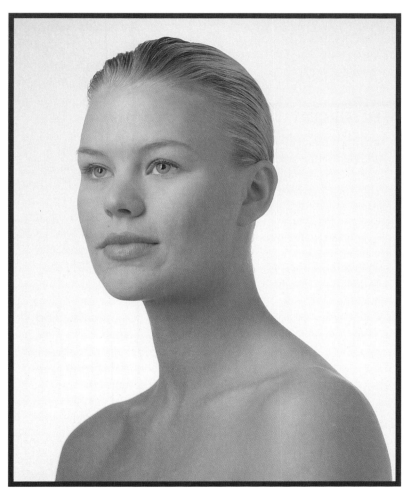

The first look often determines our first impressions. Subconsciously we have a tendency to categorize people by the texture and color of their skin.

CHAPTER

7

CHAPTER

7

Fortunately, modern medicine has provided us with the means to put into perspective many of these misconceptions.

Our agenda for a uniform complexion includes:

■ *laser surgery*
■ *dermabrasions*
■ *chemical peels*
■ *cryopeels*

LASER SURGERY

"Father Time eventually takes away what Mother Nature gives" goes the old saying. The soft full features of youth eventually give way to the aging signs of wrinkles, splotches of discoloration and the leathery texture of weathered skin.

Good basic skin care can forestall many signs of aging but of course Father Time will eventually win. Fortunately we have a weapon – the laser.

Laser technology for the treatment of skin problems has exploded over the last five years. Conditions, which could not be treated in the past without the risk of scarring, such a birthmarks and pigmented lesions, can now be removed with little or no complications. A new generation of lasers are largely responsible for this breakthrough.

Laser is an acronym for the Light Amplification by the Stimulated Emission of Radiation. Laser light is distinguished from other forms of light by two characteristics:

■ The emitted light is columnated rather than scattered. All the light goes in one direction.

■ The wave lengths of light are parallel and in phase with one another.

It is the wave length of the emitted light which distinguishes one laser from another and the way they affect the skin. For example, the Alexandrite laser (a pigment removal laser) has a different wave length than the Variable Pulse Width (VPW) laser (a vascular removal laser) which explains why they target different colors in the skin. The wavelength is determined by the substance which generates the light, for example, a ruby crystal in a Q-switched ruby laser, a red dye in a flashlamp pumped pulsed dye laser, and a carbon dioxide gas in a CO_2 laser. An electric current, radio wave, or flashlamp passes through the light generating medium stimulating the molecules to produce the laser light.

Lasers have become increasingly complex and the variations in their wave length, pulse duration, intensity of light and other parameters are important to the engineers, physicists and laser surgeons. What is important to the patient is that the advances in this technology have significantly changed the way in which many skin conditions are treated and surgeries are performed.

Lasers in dermatology are used to:

- remove discoloration (pigment and blood vessels) from the skin,

- remove growths from the skin,

- resurface the skin, and

- cut the skin.

Removal of Red Discolorations of the Skin

Port wine haemangiomas (birthmarks) are probably the most common type of vascular disorders which cause red discolorations of the skin. These blood vessel changes are usually of no medical consequence but present major cosmetic disabilities to some individuals. In the past, a person with a birthmark had the choice between living with the disorder or risking excessive scarring from surgical removal or radiation therapy. Target specific vascular lasers have essentially eliminated this risk, thereby offering many individuals a new lease on life.

The most current and advanced of the vascular lasers are the Variable Pulse Width (VPW) and the flashlamp pumped pulsed dye (Dye) lasers. The argon laser was the first vascular laser to be used. It is no longer recommended

for this purpose because there is too much heat dissipated which may result in scarring. Other vascular lasers have the same problem but to a lesser extent.

Facial veins begin to appear as we age and are largely the result of excessive sun exposure although heredity does play a role. Fine, superficial veins respond well to the Dye laser, whereas the VPW laser is often required to get rid of deeper, larger vessels. An additional benefit of the VPW laser is that it does not leave a bruise, whereas the Dye laser does.

Sclerotherapy is still the treatment of choice for leg veins, however lasers and other photothermal instruments are beginning to make inroads into this area as well. If the veins on the legs are very fine giving a blush like appearance or thick and resistant to sclerotherapy then a vascular laser such as the VPW laser may be used. Sclerotherapy and light treatments for leg veins are discussed in more detail in Chapter 15.

Benign blood vessel tumors also begin to crop up as we get older. Some people may mistake them as blemishes on their face and wonder at the appearance of large numbers of them over their torsos and limbs. They are of no medical consequence but many people like to have them removed with a vascular laser for cosmetic reasons.

The red discoloration found

Facial Telangiectasia

BEFORE

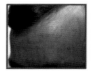

AFTER

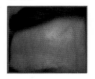

PHOTOS COURTESY OF DR. DON GROOT

CHAPTER

7

Facial Telangiectasia

BEFORE

AFTER

PHOTOS
COURTESY OF
DR. DON GROOT

in scars can also be reduced or removed with the VPW or Dye lasers, softening the cosmetic disability caused by the scar, particularly if it appears on the face.

Radiation therapy for cancer will cause dilated blood vessels to appear on the skin of the treated area. This is particularly common on the chest after radiation is used for the treatment of breast cancer. These can be removed with the VPW or Dye lasers.

How do these vascular removal lasers work?

The wave length of light that is produced by vascular removal lasers has a selective affinity for blood vessels. It passes harmlessly through the top layer or epidermis of the skin leaving it essentially intact. The VPW laser actually cools the top layer of the skin with a chilled tip through which the laser light passes. This further spares the skin from the risk of scarring and irregular pigmentation. When the light hits the targeted blood vessels it causes a microscopic fragmentations or sealing of the blood vessels. The dispersed blood cells are then carried away by the body's garbage collecting cells (macrophages) leaving behind normal skin.

Does a treatment with a vascular removal laser hurt?

The light from the laser is emitted in pulses. Each pulse feels like someone has snapped an elastic band against the skin. Most adults tolerate the discomfort from the VPW or Dye lasers very well. The chilled tip of the VPW laser reduces this discomfort considerably. Also, a new device has been designed to reduce discomfort with the pulse dye lasers. It delivers a short jet of cool gas upon the skin just prior to the laser application.

Children vary in their level of tolerance and this is usually directly proportional to how frightened they are. For adults with a low pain threshold and for children an anesthetic cream is provided. In some cases where a vascular lesion, such as a port wine hemangioma, is extensive intravenous sedation may be warranted.

How does the skin look and feel after a treatment with the vascular removal lasers?

A mild burning sensation may be experienced for up to two hours after a treatment session. This is easily controlled by an analgesic such as Tylenol. Aspirin or any other medication that contains acetylsalicylic acid should be avoided because they affect the way in which the blood clots and may encourage bruising.

CHAPTER

7

YOUNG AS YOU LOOK

The VPW laser seldom causes bruising and usually leaves a slightly pink area which fades within a couple of hours. If the lesion is deep and a greater power is used a blotchy, pink, superficial welt may occur. This disappears to normal skin an hour or two after the surgery. In some instances a crust may form.

When the Dye laser is used a deep purple discoloration of the skin similar to a bruise is evident for 7 to 12 days after a treatment session. This fades to a brown color which may take up to 6 weeks to disappear entirely.

How many treatments are required?

The number of treatment sessions depends on the size, location and depth of the lesion. For example, if a port wine hemangioma involves half the face and is very thick many sessions will be required to cover the extensive surface and to gradually remove the layers of vessels. Whereas, a small number of superficial vessels may only require one session.

Thicker vessels in vascular lesions such as cavernous hemangiomas and facial veins respond better to the VPW laser. The chilled tip allows the laser light to dwell on the vessel for a longer period of time without causing damage to the surrounding skin.

This allows the laser light to seal the vessel, eradicating the lesion.

Are vascular removal lasers safe?

Yes, the VPW and Dye lasers are safe. Because the energy from the laser beam is absorbed by the abnormal vasculature and does not affect the surrounding tissue the risk of scarring is very low. Safety goggles must be worn by the patient and the laser surgeon during the procedure to protect the eyes from the bright light.

What are the possible complications associated with vascular removal lasers?

Post-operative complications from treatment with the VPW or Dye lasers are very rare. However, with any surgery there are inherent risks. The potential adverse side effects from these lasers may include: scarring, crusting, thinning of the skin, hyperpigmentation (a brown discoloration), hypopigmentation (loss of color) or a slight depression at the treatment site.

Can anyone with a vascular lesion be treated with a vascular removal laser?

There are some people who would not be good candidates for vascular laser surgery. People who are sensitive to light due to heredity, disease or medication are not candidates for this treatment.

CHAPTER

7

Tattoo Removal

BEFORE

AFTER

PHOTOS
COURTESY OF
DR. DON GROOT

For example, seizures triggered by light or the use of blood thinning medications are contraindications for treatment with a vascular removal laser. Very dark skinned individuals tend to develop hypopigmentation (a lack of color) when treated with a vascular removal laser. This is usually temporary.

What does it cost to have vascular laser surgery of the skin?

The cost is dependent on the size, location and depth of the vascular lesion. Most dermatologic surgeons charge a facilities fee plus a per pulse charge for the laser on a session by session basis. A small lesion may cost only $200 whereas an extensive birthmark may cost $400 to $1500 per session.

Removal of Dark Discolorations of the Skin and Tattoos

Pigmented lesions which tend to be brown or black in color are caused by an excess number of pigment producing cells, known as melanocytes, in the skin. When stimulated by hormonal changes or exposure to ultraviolet light the melanocytes produce excess amounts of melanin resulting in dark discolorations of the skin. Age spots, moles, freckles, lentigos, melasma, and blue or black birthmarks known as congenital nevi are common

examples of these changes in the skin. There are a number of treatment options for these conditions which include cryo-therapy (cold therapy with liquid nitrogen), surgical removal, and bleaching creams. The Q-switched ruby, Alexandrite, and Nd:Yag lasers have provided treatment options which in some cases have significantly reduced the risk of scarring and have provided an alternative when other treatment options were ineffective.

Tattoos could be referred to as self-induced pigmented lesions of the skin. Tattoos are created when ink and other metallic particles are injected into the second layer of the skin, known as the dermis, or when dirt and other debris is embedded in the skin from a traumatic injury, such as a motorcycle accident on an asphalt surface. The latter is often called a dirt tattoo or road rash.

The methods of tattoo removal in the past frequently left unsightly scars. These include resurfacing techniques, such as salabrasion (salt scraping), dermabrasion (mechanical sanding), and chemical peels, as well as surgical techniques such as skin grafting. With the advent of the pigment removal lasers the risk of scarring has been significantly reduced and the results are cosmetically superior.

All the pigment removal lasers are useful for removing black and blue ink from tattoos. However if a tattoo is complex in

CHAPTER

7

YOUNG AS YOU LOOK

color and variety then it is more difficult to remove. Utilizing a combination of the pigment removal lasers most of the colors in a multi-colored tattoo can be removed as each of the wavelengths of light tends to have an affinity for slightly different ranges of colors. It is very expensive for most laser surgeons to own all three types of pigment removal lasers. Recognizing this Coherent Medical Group produced a laser with three wavelengths of light, the Versapulse Integrated Laser System. This has allowed the laser surgeon to remove not only blacks but reds, greens, and yellows from tattoos.

How do the pigment removal lasers work?

The pigment removal lasers work in a similar fashion to the vascular lasers. The intense light from the laser passes harmlessly through the top layer of the skin and is selectively absorbed by colored pigment particles within the skin. The pigment cells or the ink of a tattoo break into minuscule particles which are removed by the body's immune system.

Does a treatment with a pigment removal laser hurt?

The light from the lasers is emitted in pulses. Each pulse feels like someone has snapped an elastic band against the skin. These pulses

are emitted at different speeds in different lasers. Both children and adults vary in their level of pain tolerance. An anesthetic cream may be provided for adults with a low pain threshold and for children.

How does the skin look and feel after a treatment with a pigment removal laser?

Each pulse of the laser light leaves the targeted skin altered in appearance. It may be slightly grey or red in color. Some bleeding or blistering may occur and is more common with the Nd:Yag laser, than the Alexandrite and Q-switched ruby lasers. Within minutes the treatment site turns to a dark, superficial crust. The crust remains until the top layer of the skin turns over, leaving a pale, pink, smooth surface. The length of time it takes for the crust to be sloughed depends on the type of condition being treated and where on the body it occurs. For example, the crusting of an age spot on the face will turn over faster than one on the back of the hand. On average, the process takes one to two weeks. The new, underlying skin will gradually change from a pink shade to the color of the surrounding skin within a couple of weeks.

Are pigment removal lasers safe?

Yes, these lasers are safe. Special eye protection must be worn by both

Road Rash

BEFORE

AFTER

PHOTOS COURTESY OF DR. DON GROOT

CHAPTER

7

BEFORE

AFTER

the patient and the laser surgeon during the procedure to protect the eyes from the bright light.

What complications may occur?

A potential complication with this procedure is hypopigmentation where the treated area ends up being lighter than the surrounding tissue. This risk is higher in darker skinned individuals.

The risk of scarring is very low because the laser light is absorbed by the targeted pigment leaving the surrounding tissue relatively untouched. Infection is rare.

Permanent coloration is a tattooing technique which has recently become popular for the enhancement of facial features such as the eyebrows, eyes and lips. Pigments used in permanent coloration often contain iron. When the laser light hits these pigments it alters the color causing them to become black. Rather than

laser removal to correct or remove permanent makeup a more effective technique is to tattoo tannic acid into the unwanted color which causes it to gradually bleach out.

How many treatments are required and what will it cost?

The number of treatment sessions depends on the size, location, depth and color of the pigmented lesion or tattoo. These factors also determine the cost.

Superficial lesions such as age spots usually require fewer sessions than a deeper lesion such as congenital nevi or decorative tattoos. The latter often requires a layered approach.

Treatment sessions are spaced 3 to 6 weeks apart. This allows the garbage collecting cells of the immune system to gather up the maximum amount of left over pigment between each session.

Resurfacing Techniques

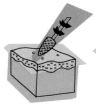

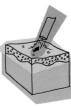

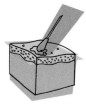

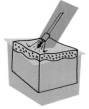

DERMABRASION   LASER RESURFACING   CHEMICAL PEEL   CRYO-PEEL

CHAPTER

7

RESURFACING TECHNIQUES

Resurfacing is a term which encompasses several different surgical techniques; laser resurfacing, dermabrasion, chemical peeling and cryotherapy. Through different modalities each of these techniques removes the superficial layer of the skin (epidermis and upper portion of the dermis), followed by its regeneration. The regenerated skin is also rejuvenated, we therefore see a reduction of sun-induced wrinkles, better skin tone, and a uniformity of color and texture.

Mechanical dermabrasion and chemical peeling with phenol or trichloroacetic acid have been used for many years. Laser resurfacing is relatively new and provides many advantages over the traditional approaches including a lower risk of scarring, less post-operative pain, a shorter healing time, and more uniform results.

Laser Resurfacing For Wrinkles, Irregular Pigmentation and Scar

The carbon dioxide laser may be used in a focused mode for cutting or a defocussed mode for vaporizing the skin. In the cutting mode it is used in delicate surgical techniques such as eyelid correction. The advantage is that as the laser cuts it seals off the blood vessels and nerve endings which decreases the time for healing and the amount of post-operative pain.

In the vaporizing mode the carbon dioxide (CO_2) laser is used to remove abnormal tissue such as warts and scars and more recently to resurface the skin to stimulate rejuvenation.

The wavelength of the CO_2 laser heats the cells of the unwanted skin or abnormal tissue to the point where it is vaporized away in a plume of tissue particles and steam. If the heat is excessive there is a risk of scarring or pigment changes to the adjacent normal skin tissue.

When the CO_2 laser was first introduced as a surgical tool the light was delivered continuously to the skin. This was only interrupted when the surgeon released the foot pedal to close the shutter and prevent the escape of the laser light beam. The control over the dissipation of heat was poor and the risk of damage was high. It took a highly skilled surgeon to judge what power and time duration of laser light would remove abnormal tissue without damaging the surrounding tissue. For this reason the use of the CO_2 laser as a surgical tool was relatively uncommon for a number of years and when it was used it was reserved for the removal or alteration of abnormal tissue, such as warts.

Laser Resurfacing of Wrinkles

BEFORE

AFTER

PHOTOS COURTESY OF DR. DON GROOT

CHAPTER

7

Developments in CO_2 laser technology have focused on controlling the heat produced by the laser light so that only targeted tissue is affected. The UltraPulse and TruTouch CO_2 lasers have accomplished this by computerized delivery of extremely short repetitive pulses. The time in between each pulse allows the skin to cool so that the heat does not remain in the tissue long enough to cause more damage than is intended. Other lasers, such as the Silk Touch CO_2 laser, have achieved the necessary control over heat dissipation by moving the continuous wave of laser light around very rapidly so it does not dwell in any one area for very long. This is also controlled by computer.

Both types of technology seem to be effective in controlling heat transfer. The deciding factor in the outcome of CO_2 laser surgery and especially resurfacing is the skill of the surgeon. Despite testimonials to the contrary, computerized controlled delivery of the laser light cannot do all the work. The laser is the brush and the surgeon is the artist. If a surgeon simply moves the laser light over the surface of the skin obliterating everything in its path then the healing process will be slow and the results less than satisfactory.

What is involved in laser resurfacing?

The Step in Facial Surgery (Chapter 8) apply to laser resurfacing with some qualifications.

Prior to laser resurfacing the regular use of topical creams containing tretinoin and/or glycolic acid for 6 weeks or more is recommended by some surgeons to prepare the skin for the surgery. It is also common for patients who have a history of herpes cold sores to begin taking an anti-viral medication such as Valtrex to prevent the eruption and spread of a cold sore in response to the resurfacing.

A local anesthetic or nerve block is administered so no pain is experienced during the procedure. For more extensive areas, such as a full face laser resurfacing for wrinkles and scars, an intravenous or general anesthetic may be recommended.

The eyes are protected from the bright laser beam with special goggles. If the surgeon plans to go in close proximity to the eye then a protective shield is placed over the eye. The eye is anesthetized with drops and the shield is covered with a lubricant prior to putting it in place.

The best results are achieved when a combination of free hand and computerized controlled delivery are used. Free hand places the power and duration of the laser light into the hands of the surgeon, allowing precise removal of irregularities and contour deformities in the skin. The surgeon outlines a surgical plan in permanent ink on the scars or wrinkles to be resurfaced. Using the freehand modality the targeted irregularities in the skin are removed. The computerized controlled delivery is then employed to blend the edges of the areas treated with the free hand modality and to resurface more uniform skin. This also evens out irregularities in pigmentation.

The free hand approach allows the surgeon control over the results but also requires that the surgeon is highly skilled. If a surgeon simply uses the computerized controlled delivery unnecessary tissue is lost and the time required for healing takes longer. However, if a surgeon does not understand how the tissue responds to the laser and does not recognize the subtle changes in the tissue when the laser light interacts with the skin, then they are better off using the computerized controlled delivery alone.

After the resurfacing is complete the treated area may be covered with dressings or left open at the discretion of the surgeon. The use of a dressing hides the raw, oozing skin and may help to reduce post-operative discomfort. Flexan or Silon II are the most commonly used dressings. Flexan does not allow for careful visual observation of the skin for potential infection and other complications because it is opaque. Silon II is clear. If dressings are used they are left in place for 1 to 7 days.

Does the procedure hurt?

Anesthetic is used to avoid any discomfort during the procedure.

The amount of pain experienced after the procedure depends on the extent of the procedure. Any discomfort may be controlled with painkillers such as Tylenol. Acetylsalicylic acid (Aspirin) is not recommended as bruising may be encouraged.

How should the face look after laser resurfacing?

The treated skin is dry and blanched (white) immediately after the application of the laser light. The surgeon wipes this debris away and the underlying skin is very red.

The first few days after surgery can be quite alarming to the patient, if a full face laser resurfacing is performed, especially if the face is not covered with semi-occlusive dressings. The face often becomes very swollen and gooey (Appendix: Patient Diary).

The skin passes through three phases of healing over the course of 10 to 14 days:

Oozing /Crusting Phase

During the initial healing phase oozing and less often a crust or scab will develop over the treatment site. If a dressing is applied then the following regime is not necessary. Many people find the semi-occlusive dressings annoying after the first couple of days and would like the opportunity to cleanse their skin.

If a dressing is not applied it is important to keep the skin well

CHAPTER

7

lubricated and prevent drying until the oozing has stopped. This is usually accomplished with big gobs of petroleum jelly (Vaseline) or Aquaphor. As distasteful as this sounds it is the most effective way of trapping the moisture in the skin and preventing it from drying and cracking.

An antibiotic ointment such as Fucidin ointment will have been applied immediately after the surgery. Some physicians suggest that their patients continue to apply this under the moisturizer, although it can be irritating for some people.

During the crusting phase the face should be cleansed with very cold water and a mild cleanser such as Neutrogena or Pears. For the first 2 days this is a challenge because the water feels like a million little pin pricks on the face. Rather than splashing the water on the face a sterile gauze is recommended to gently pat the area with the cleanser and water.

Serum literally drips down the face during the first 2 to 3 days. Gently wiping the serum away frequently with a cold, wet, sterile gauze and reapplying the moisturizer helps the skin to feel more comfortable.

Extensive swelling during the first 3 days is common with full face resurfacing. It can be disconcerting to look in the mirror and not recognize yourself because of the distortion to your facial features. The surgeon may opt to give a dose of cortisone either through injection or tablets to reduce the swelling.

The treatment site usually looks worse than it feels but acetaminophen (Tylenol) may be recommended to control discomfort. Oral antibiotics and anti-viral cold sore medications, such as Valtrex, are rarely required but are often used prophylactically.

If crusts form they will begin to separate from the skin within a week, although on some areas of the face this may take longer. It is important that the crusts are not picked or dislodged as this may lead to scarring. They will drop off when they are ready.

Towards the end of the oozing and crusting phase the skin becomes very itchy, as the skin heals. The regular application of cold water and petroleum jelly helps to control the desire to itch as does the use of an antihistamine such as Reactine.

Flaky Phase

Once the oozing stops or any crusts have been sloughed there will be a period of flakiness for several days during which desquamated (dead) skin comes loose. During this phase the skin should continue to be well lubricated using Aquaphor, Vaseline or a moisturizer, such as Moisturel Cream after gentle cleansing.

Signs of hyperpigmentation develop during this stage in some patients. The skin begins to turn a blotchy brown color. Within 2 months this disappears although it is worthwhile to encourage resolution of hyperpigmentation with bleaching creams.

Sun exposure should be avoided as much as possible. Protection with a broad spectrum sunscreen, such as Ombrelle lotion with an SPF of 15 or more is essential in order to prevent a severe eruption of hyperpigmentation.

Erythema (Pink) Phase

The new skin will be very red at first, then it will gradually fade to pink, then to the color of normal skin. This phase may last from 3 to 6 months. Some physicians claim that Cellex C, a vitamin C preparation, helps to reduce the redness and shorten the length of this phase.

It is important to avoid rubbing the skin, to apply moisturizers liberally and to protect the skin from sun exposure. Makeup may be used once all the flakiness has disappeared.

If the post-operative red discoloration is mild, an ordinary base makeup will probably be adequate. An opaque makeup is useful when the pinkness is quite intense.

For deeper, red erythema it may be necessary to use a green base foundation under the cream base concealer. This neutralizes the red discoloration.

It is essential to protect the treated skin from the sun with broad spectrum sunscreens, sun hats and sunglasses. If this is not done hyperpigmentation is likely to occur and the skin will become a mottled brown color.

When can normal activities be resumed?

Normal social activities and work may be resumed once the scabs have fallen off (in 10 to 14 days), even though the skin is still quite red. The redness may last for 3 to 6 months.

What complications may occur?

The potential problems associated with laser resurfacing are:

- **Scarring:** Problematic scarring may result, but rarely occurs when the surgery is performed by an experienced surgeon. When it does occur it is usually due to an inherited tendency for excessive scarring or may be due to the laser light having penetrated too deeply.

- **Acne/Perioral Dermatitis:** After laser resurfacing the oil gland openings are temporarily swollen and prone to blockage. If we add to this the occlusion of a dressing, petroleum jelly and other topical preparations, acne and/or perioral dermatitis, wherein the glands become inflamed, may occur. These conditions are readily treated

CHAPTER

7

with medications that open the pores, cleanse them and allow ongoing drainage. Usually topical mixtures of mild cortisone and antibiotics suffice, but oral antibiotics may be required. Strong cortisone mixtures actually worsen the problem if used for more than a very brief interval. Here is where "reading the skin's needs" is crucial to resolution of the problem and dermatologic experience is essential for successful resolution of these complications.

- **Pigmentation Change:** Altered pigmentation may occur. This depends on the depth of the laser resurfacing, the color of the patient's skin, and the unpredictable nature of repigmentation and rejuvenation of the skin.

- **Milia:** Tiny, white cysts are rare, but may occur. They are easily removed with electrodesiccation or the CO_2 laser.

- **Other problems:** Although rare, infection, persistent redness, and a lack of response to the treatment may occur.

What else is new in laser resurfacing?

The Erbium Yag laser has recently been introduced as a resurfacing laser. It does not penetrate as deeply into the skin as the carbon dioxide lasers and is beneficial for the removal of superficial wrinkles and pigment changes. If performed as a light superficial peel, topical anesthetic creams may be all that is necessary for pain control. Reports suggest that patients heal faster and experience less redness because there is not as much heat transfer into the skin. Multiple serial sessions may be necessary to reach an acceptable end point. Time will tell where the Erbium Yag laser fits among the current options available for skin rejuvenation.

Who performs laser resurfacing and what is the cost?

Esthetic surgeons with backgrounds in dermatology and plastic surgery who are trained in laser surgery perform laser resurfacing. Here we must strongly suggest that the consumer beware. There are many physicians beginning to perform laser resurfacing who have no knowledge of the skin nor do they have surgical training or experience. These physicians believe that the laser will do all the work and they simply have to point and shoot. Such an approach will not provide optimum results and may lead to unexpected and alarming complications.

The cost varies with the number of sessions required, the extent of the surgery, and the physician's geographic location, skill, and experience. A partial face laser resurfacing may cost from $1,200 to $2,000 and a full face from $2,500 to $5,000.

DERMABRASION

When the term dermabrasion is used, it generally refers to abrasive or mechanical dermabrasion rather than laser dermabrasion, which is more often called laser resurfacing or lasabrasion. An abrasive dermabrasion literally sands down the skin with a rotating wire brush or diamond drill, whereas laser resurfacing utilizes a powerful light which heats up individual cells to 100° centigrade and vaporizes them. Lasers are rapidly replacing dermabrasions as a resurfacing technique because the results are more reliable, the laser is more versatile and the post-operative healing time is shorter and less traumatic.

Dermabrasions are classified according to the depth of the procedure. Superficial dermabrasions, also referred to as epidermal dermabrasions or epiabrasions, sand only the top layer of the skin. Deeper dermabrasions enter the second layer of the skin and are usually referred to simply as dermabrasions.

Who would benefit from a dermabrasion?

An abrasive dermabrasion is usually reserved for patients with thick, heavy skin who have experienced a loss of elasticity due to acne scarring or wrinkling. Finer skin, on the other hand, often does better with chemical peels. Laser resurfacing tends to be more versatile, and is equally good for both thick and fine skin.

Mechanical dermabrasions are not effective for removing fine, dilated blood vessels on the face. A vascular removal laser is necessary for this purpose. In some cases a dermabrasion may be used to even out irregular pigmentation, remove scaly, pre-cancerous spots, and reshape thickened noses.

Dermabrasion, however, will not totally eliminate these problems in all cases. Usually, a superficial dermabrasion will rid the skin of problems such as irregular pigment-ation that tend to occur on the surface. Deeper scars and wrinkles cannot be entirely obliterated without entering the deeper layers of the skin. This increases the risk of excessive scarring and the development, rather than reduction of, pigment irregularities.

What is involved in a dermabrasion?

The table Steps in Facial Surgery in Chapter 8 applies to mechanical dermabrasions with the following variations:

- Test sites of approximately 2 centimeters (3/4 of an inch) in diameter are carried out in front of the ear or along the temple. The test provides some idea of potential problems that may result with a complete dermabrasion and therefore

CHAPTER

7

assists in deciding whether or not to proceed. If only small areas are to be resurfaced, a test is not always necessary.

■ Superficial dermabrasions may be preceded by three weeks to three months of tretinoin application in the belief that the skin will heal faster. If the patient has a history of cold sores (which may be activated by the surgery) they are given a course of anti-viral medication, such as Valtrex, orally before and after surgery to decrease the risk of the cold sore spreading into the abraded areas.

■ A local anesthetic is injected. Then ice, artificial ice bags or cold sprays, are applied to the skin for 15 minutes prior to the sanding procedure. This helps make the skin rigid and therefore easier to sand.

■ The skin is sanded in segments and the duration of the procedure varies according to the speed of the surgeon, the extent and depth of the sanding, and the patient's cooperation. A full face derma-brasion may last between 10 and 45 minutes. The sound of the whirling burr is similar to a dentist's drill.

■ Deeper dermabrasions leave the skin raw, red, and seeping immediately after the procedure. Blood-clotting agents as well as an antibiotic ointment such as Fucidin or antibiotic soaked gauzes such as Fucidin Intertulle are often applied to the skin. The skin is then covered with surgical dressings. Special surgical dressings are sometimes used to encourage rejuvenation of the epidermis (top layer of the skin). Use of these new dressings is of particular benefit because they do not stick, causing less discomfort for the patient. Healing is faster and thick crusts are less likely to occur, but it is uncertain that any of these surgical dressings improve the cosmetic result.

What will the skin look like after dermabrasion?

A superficial dermabrasion does not improve deep wrinkles and scars but removes fine wrinkles and leaves the skin with a healthy glow. The scab usually falls off within 5 days of the procedure. The underlying skin is pink in color and gradually fades to a normal skin tone over several weeks.

Deeper dermabrasions initially leave the face red and raw. This is followed by a swollen, scabby phase. The scabs generally take 10 to 14 days to fall off. The final phase of healing is characterized by an initial period of redness which gradually fades to a normal skin tone over a 3 to 6 month period.

Does a dermabrasion hurt?

The procedure itself does not hurt because the area is anesthetized.

CHAPTER

7

118   *Y O U N G   A S   Y O U   L O O K*

Once the anesthetic wears off, however, moderate discomfort will be experienced which can be managed with painkillers. Aspirin should not be used because it may encourage bleeding.

What care should be taken after dermabrasion?

It is important the patient receives detailed instructions for the post-operative period. These basic steps are outlined in the table on the Steps in Facial Surgery in Chapter 8. Some precautionary measures specific to the dermabrasions are necessary.

If swelling and inflammation occur, cortisone may be prescribed. The skin's healing process must be monitored as infection may lead to scarring.

Once the scabs are off, the face is usually very red. As long as the abraded area is dry, makeup may be used, though cautiously. Avoidance of direct or strong sunlight, as well as the use of sun hats and broad spectrum sunscreens, is absolutely necessary for 6 months after a dermabrasion since irregular pigmentation from sun exposure may lead to skin mottling. Sunscreens should be worn thereafter to protect the rejuvenated skin.

When can normal activities be resumed?

During the first week after a deep dermabrasion the patient will be physically and cosmetically disabled because of the discomfort and swelling of the wound. When the scab forms within a week, most of the discomfort will have subsided. Patients generally feel comfortable returning to work and their normal social activities once the scabs fall off within 2 or 3 weeks, although the skin is quite red initially. This process is shorter with superficial dermabrasions and normal activities can usually be resumed after one week.

Can a dermabrasion be combined with other techniques?

Dermabrasion is often performed along with chemical peeling. The eyelid area, for example, may be peeled chemically, whereas the thicker areas of skin may be dermabraded. This blends the edges of the dermabrasion into the thinner skin of the eyes, thereby avoiding obvious demarcations. Collagen implants may be used after dermabrasion to elevate deeper depressions. Prior to a dermabrasion, a punch-transplant technique may be used on deep "ice-pick" scars. The dermabrasion will smooth out the irregularities of the punch-transplant.

What complications can occur?

Complications may occur after mechanical dermabrasions including the usual reactions such as allergies to medications or infection. The most common

CHAPTER

7

complications in order of frequency are as follows:

■ *Scarring due to:*

Excessive freezing of the skin prior to the dermabrasion.

Inadvertent gouging of deeper tissue, leaving a trough in the skin.

Accidental damage to the skin due to mishaps with the machinery.

A predisposition for excessive scarring in certain locations on the face. Darker skinned individuals are more prone to this.

Infection.

■ *Altered pigmentation:*
A loss of color in the skin (hypopigmentation) rather than an increase is more likely to occur after dermabrasion. This is because pigment cells in the skin's top layer may either be destroyed during the cold applications prior to dermabrasion or removed during the procedure.

If the dermabrasion is deep, pigment cells around the hair sheaths will also be affected. Skin irritation on the other hand, may cause stimulation of pigment cells resulting in the production of more melanin and a darker color to the abraded area (hyperpigmentation). Individuals with dark skin are more prone to a mottled or

uneven complexion after dermabrasion. This is particularly true if they are exposed to too much ultraviolet light in the post-operative period.

Skin color changes present cosmetic problems, particularly for men. Women feel comfortable using cover-up makeup but this might seem too "feminine" for some men.

■ *Milia:* Tiny oil-gland cysts may appear during the healing period because the oil glands cannot drain properly. The gland breaks under the skin and the body's defences cause a small wall to form around it resulting in milia. They will usually disappear spontaneously. They also could be obliterated quickly with gentle, electro-desiccation, laser therapy or a small incision may be used to open the skin over the tiny white cyst.

■ *Other potential problems:*
The trauma of dermabrasion may aggravate underlying disorders such as acne, lupus erythematosus, or cold sore infections. A poor result, persistent redness, or the development of telangiectasia are also potential problems.

Who performs dermabrasions and what do they cost?

Dermatologists and plastic surgeons usually perform dermabrasions, but other physicians and surgeons may be trained in this procedure. It is up to the patient to ask their physician about his or her qualifications and training.

The cost varies with the number of sessions necessary, the amount of skin treated, the geographic location of the physician, and the skill and experience of the operator. Generally, a partial face dermabrasion costs from $200 to $800 and a full face dermabrasion $800 to $1800.

CHEMICAL PEELS

Chemical peels have been used in France since the late nineteenth century to combat skin aging. They have been used in North America since the 1920s, and are now accepted and well recognized procedures, particularly for treatment of sun damaged and aged skin.

A variety of chemical agents are used to cause inflammation and irritation to the superficial layers of the skin. Three of the most commonly used peeling agents are phenol and its derivatives, trichloroacetic acid, and alpha hydroxy acids. The subsequent realignment of the skin's collagen building blocks after the chemical peel leads to a smoother, younger look.

What benefits can a chemical peel yield?

Sun damaged skin characterized by fine to moderately coarse wrinkles, irregular pigmentation, dilated blood vessels, and scaling would all benefit from a chemical peel. Light skinned patients are better candidates than those with darker skin because they tend to have fewer pigmentation problems, such as a blotchy color, after the procedure. Individuals with sagging and excessive skin are not candidates for this procedure, since chemical peeling improves skin quality but does not reduce excess skin. An eyelid lift, for example, removes redundant skin, but chemical peeling may be necessary to remove the fine wrinkles.

What is involved in a chemical peel?

Chemical peels can be categorized as mild, moderate and aggressive. The extent of skin damage determines the type of peel which is used and the depth of peeling necessary.

Mild chemical peels: A solution of 30 to 70% glycolic acid or 10 to 15% trichloroacetic acid may be used.

Moderate chemical peels: 20 to 45% trichloroacetic acid is used.

Aggressive peels: 45 to 60% trichloroacetic acid, phenol, or Baker's solution (a modified phenol preparation) may be used.

Many dermatologists, plastic surgeons, and other esthetic surgeons are now using milder agents in a series of applications

CHAPTER

7

rather than using more aggressive agents on a single occasion to obtain the best results with the least amount of risk.

The glycolic acid peels are particularly popular because they offer the least risk of pigment changes and scar, as well as the shortest period of cosmetic disability after the procedure. In contrast, with the phenol peels there is a greater risk of scar and pigment changes, a longer recovery time, and the risk of damage to the heart, liver and kidneys.

The steps involved with each type of peel are similar, with some differences:

- If phenol is used for the peeling procedure, a pre-operative assessment of the heart, liver, and kidneys is necessary. This is not necessary with glycolic acid and trichloroacetic acid peels.

- With all types of peels, the skin is cleaned with degreasing agents, such as acetone, alcohol, or povidone-iodine (Betadine), as these encourage better penetration to deeper levels and greater uniformity of the peel.

- The chemical agent of choice is usually applied with Q-Tips or gauze over the designated areas. Feathering, using less or lower concentrations of the agent, is performed as the physician moves from the face into the neck or hairline regions. This avoids any

obvious demarcation between peeled and untreated skin.

- Different techniques may be used. For example, with the Jessner technique a mild peeling solution may be applied prior to a stronger solution in order to remove the epidermis. This allows the second solution (either glycolic or trichloroacetic acid) to reach the dermis immediately minimizing the amount of time it has to be left on the skin. With the Obaji and other techniques the patient is required to use a variety of creams containing tretinoin and other agents prior to the chemical peel in order to prepare the skin to be chemically resurfaced.

Phenol preparations, such as Baker's formula, penetrate deeper than do other agents and can be absorbed into the body, causing internal damage. Strict time parameters must, therefore, be observed. This controlled absorption minimizes the risk of damage to the heart, liver, or kidneys. The heart must be monitored for irregularities throughout the procedure when phenol solutions are used.

- The skin may blanch when an agent is applied. This is commonly called "frosting" and means that chemical coagulation of the deeper layers of the skin has occurred. Not all areas of the face blanch at the same rate; thin and sensitive areas blanch faster than others. For this reason, the surgeon may apply stronger concentrations of the agent to areas of thicker skin, such as the forehead while minimizing the amount of agent applied to thin, sensitive areas, such as the eyelids, by using a lower concentration.

- The time needed to apply an agent to the entire face may range from a matter of minutes to 2 hours depending on which agents are used. More aggressive peels take longer.

- The chemical is neutralized with cold water once the required effect has been achieved.

- Post-operative care is similar to that for other resurfacing techniques.

Does a chemical peel hurt?

The patient should be prepared for some discomfort while the chemical is being applied, particularly with more aggressive agents. The pain often disappears within seconds or minutes but may return later, though with less intensity.

Initially, the pain varies in intensity from mild to moderate and is often replaced by itching during the healing process. The itching usually subsides after the scabs have come off, although it may persist in some cases. Sensations of warmth and tightness are also experienced after a chemical peel.

What will the face look like after a chemical peel?

The extent of cosmetic disability after a peel depends on the depth of the peel. Superficial, or "freshening peels," using lower chemical concentrations cause mild inflammation and swelling which softens the appearance of wrinkles for a short period of time and may lighten blotchy areas of pigment on the skin.

Higher concentrations of trichloroacetic acid or of alpha hydroxy acids, such as glycolic acid, will result in redness, swelling, and, in some cases, oozing. Peeling and crusting (if oozing occurs) normally disappear within 5 to 7 days. The underlying skin is light pink and gradually fades to normal skin color over a period of several weeks. For some patients, a series of moderate peels provides the best results while minimizing the risk factor.

Deeper peels, using higher concentrations of trichloroacetic acid and phenol or its derivatives, cause swelling and oozing of clear or yellowish serum. A scab then forms and is usually sloughed off in 10 to 21 days. The remaining skin is quite red and gradually fades to pink over a 3 to 6 month period.

When can normal activities be resumed?

After surgery, bed rest with the head elevated is recommended for more aggressive peels. If a large area is

SKIN REJUVENATION TECHNIQUES

Technique	Potential benefit	Potential problems
LASER SURGERY:		
Carbon Dioxide Laser and Erbium Yag Laser	Rejuvenates skin (fewer wrinkles and greater elasticity). Very low risk of scarring. Less pain and swelling. Can be used on coarse or fine skin.	Scarring. Irregular pigmentation. Prolonged erythema. Results dependent on type of carbon dioxide laser used and skill of the operator.
VPW and Pulse Dye Lasers	Removes red discolorations of the skin (blood vessels). Very low risk of scarring.	Scarring.
Q-switched Ruby, Alexandrite and Nd:Yag Lasers	Removes dark discolorations of the skin. Low risk of pigment loss or scar.	Scarring. Irregular pigmentation.

Condition to be treated	Recovery
Coarse and fine skin with scarring, wrinkles, uneven pigment and/or texture changes. Sun damaged skin with scaly spots and fine blood vessels.	10-14 days for initial healing and 3-6 months for persistent hyper-pigmentation and erythema.
Birthmarks. Facial veins (telangiectasia). Leg vein blushes. Recalcitrant leg veins. Cherry angiomas.	Immediate to 2 weeks.
Tattoos. Age spots and melasma. Blue-black birthmarks.	1-3 weeks.

CHAPTER

7

SKIN REJUVENATION TECHNIQUES

Technique	Potential benefit
DERMABRASION:	Rejuvenates thick, heavy skin (fewer wrinkles and greater elasticity).
	Beneficial for acne-scarred skin.
CHEMICAL PEELS: Chemical peel with Phenol and Derivatives	Good for marked skin damage and wrinkles.
Chemical peel with Trichloroacetic Acid	Less aggressive than phenol.
	Lower risk than phenol peels.
	Solution strengths can be tailored to the patient's needs.
Chemical peel with Alpha Hydroxy Acids (Glycolic Acid)	Good for very fine wrinkles.
	Lower risk than phenol and tricholoroacetic acid peels.
	Various acids and concentrations allow for versatility, low potency and low risk.
CRYOPEEL:	Low risk if performed regularly, cautiously and in small doses.
	Much higher risk when used as a deep peeling agent.

Potential problems	Condition to be treated	Recovery
Scarring. Irregular pigmentation. Prolonged uncomfortable healing time.	Coarser wrinkles accompanied by acne scarring and loss of elasticity. Sun damaged skin with scaly spots.	3-6 weeks for initial healing and 3 to 6 months for redness.
Scarring. Irregular pigmentation. Potential toxic effects on heart, kidneys and/or liver.	Skin with marked wrinkling and sun damage.	3-6 weeks.
Scarring. Irregular pigmentation. Different concentrations give different results.	Marked wrinkling and sun damage.	2-5 weeks.
Scarring. Irregular pigmentation.	Fine wrinkles and uneven skin color.	1 hour to 3 weeks.
Scarring. Irregular pigmentation. Requires a skilled operator. Response may be unpredictable.	Superficial sun damage. Scaly precancerous spots.	1-3 weeks.

treated, 48 hours of bed rest is required. Normal activities at home may be resumed, but a return to work and social life is not advised until after the crusts have fallen off (5 to 21 days depending on the type of peel).

What complications may occur with chemical peels?

- **Scarring:** Of the complications that may occur, scarring is the most common and cosmetically debilitating. Scarring occurs more often with deeper than with superficial peels, particularly over the angle of the jaw and around the mouth. This scarring may result in a band around the mouth resembling a purse string with gathered folds. Older skin takes longer to heal than does younger skin, but may actually scar less. Generally, darker skin has a greater risk of scar formation and irregular pigmentation.

- **Hypopigmentation:** Another complication is hypopigmentation, or loss of color, particularly with deeper peels. The opposite effect, hyperpigmentation, or too much color, may also occur and is more often seen with superficial peels.

- **Infection:** Secondary bacterial infection or activation of herpes simplex (cold sores) is a potential problem in the areas peeled. As with other forms of resurfacing, many physicians provide anti-viral medications, such as Valtrex prophylactically.

- **Toxicity:** Internal toxicity is a potential risk with phenol agents causing damage to the heart, liver, or kidneys. Trichloroacetic acid and glycolic acid (an alpha hydroxy acid) are not toxic.

Who performs chemical peels?

Dermatologists, plastic surgeons, and esthetic surgeons perform mild to aggressive chemical peels depending on the needs of the patient.

Estheticians have recently begun to perform mild chemical peels which give a fresher appearance to the skin but do not dramatically alter the color, texture and wrinkles of the skin. Unfortunately there are no standards for training or experience for estheticians performing these mild peels. It would be important to query an esthetician as to their training, competence, and experience in this area. It would also be wise to ask about the strength and type of chemical being used as well as the potential complications. Generally speaking if complications do occur estheticians are usually not trained to recognize and correct the problem before significant damage occurs.

Although the peels performed by estheticians are less expensive than those done by medically trained surgeons they are also less effective. The balance is between risk and benefit.

CHAPTER

7

YOUNG AS YOU LOOK

What does a chemical peel cost?

The cost depends on the physician's geographic location, the extent and type of peel performed, and whether general anesthetic and monitoring in an operating suite is necessary. Mild serial peels may cost from $50 to $100 per session while more aggressive peels may cost $800 to $3,000.

CRYOPEELS

Cryotherapy has been used for many years by dermatologists for the removal of age spots and other types of brown pigmented lesions from the skin. Recently it has been introduced as a full face peeling agent for the treatment of sun damaged skin.

Nitrogen in its liquid form is very cold and when sprayed on the skin will cause a localized frostbite to the top layer of the skin. This is known as cryotherapy (cold therapy).

The steps involved in a cryopeel are as follows:

- A local or topical anesthetic may be used. If a topical anesthetic is used, it may also be enhanced by other forms of painkillers and muscle relaxants. This is important as the procedure is quite painful. Some physicians use a nonsteroidal anti-inflammatory agent to help control pain.

- The skin is cleaned and the face is divided into treatment segments with a marking pen.

- The skin in each segment is stretched so the liquid nitrogen can be applied evenly to the surface of each area.

- The liquid nitrogen is sprayed onto each segment in a back and forth motion similar to the strokes of a paintbrush. If age spots are encountered more liquid nitrogen is administered to the spots in a spiral like fashion to increase the depth of destruction.

- The skin blanches when the liquid nitrogen is first applied. This is followed by a period of swelling, blistering and oozing which lasts approximately 5 days. Subsequent crusting peels off within 10 days.

- Once the peeling process is complete the skin is pink in color. This gradually fades to a normal skin tone over a period of 3 to 6 months.

Some physicians will do several very superficial cryopeels where the face is gently sprayed frequently over a period of several months. This does not get rid of age spots but does cause superficial swelling which puffs up the fine wrinkles. There is some speculation that this process may provide long term benefit by realigning the collagen in the second layer of the skin. Blistering and oozing does not occur with this technique. The skin simply feels tingly when sprayed

CHAPTER

7

and may be a bit pink for a short time afterwards.

Does cryopeeling hurt?

The initial contact of the liquid nitrogen with the skin is intensely painful, unless a nerve block or local anesthetic has been used. Premedication with a nonsteroidal anti-inflammatory agent reduces this intense pain to seconds after which the patient experiences a dull aching sensation followed by a painless throbbing which lasts approximately half an hour. Any further post-operative discomfort is easily managed with over the counter painkillers, although as with other types of surgery acetylsalicylic acid (aspirin) is not recommended.

What will the face look like after a cryopeel?

The swelling, blistering, and oozing which follows the procedure can be quite unsightly for up to 5 days. Subsequent crusting is sloughed over the next 5 day period, after which the skin appears pink and smooth and feels tighter. Most people take 2 weeks off work because of the post-operative period of cosmetic disability.

What complications may occur?

The complications that may occur with cryopeels are similar to those of other resurfacing techniques and include:

- **Pigmentary problems:** Uneven application of the liquid nitrogen may result in a blotchy appearance to the skin. Damage to the pigment producing cells, known as melanocytes, could cause hypopigmentation. Hyperpigmentation might follow inflammatory damage.

- **Scarring:** Overzealous use of the liquid nitrogen may cause damage deep into the second layer of skin which could result in scarring.

- **Infection:** As with all forms of surgery this is a rare but potential complication.

Who performs cryopeels?

Deep cryopeels are not very common because some of the other resurfacing techniques discussed, especially laser resurfacing, provide a better result with less pain and a shorter healing time. Superficial cryopeels are more common and are used to freshen the skin and remove age spots. Dermatologists or other esthetic surgeons trained in the technique would perform cryopeels.

CHAPTER

7

YOUNG AS YOU LOOK

The *Face & Neck*

AN UPLIFTING EXPERIENCE

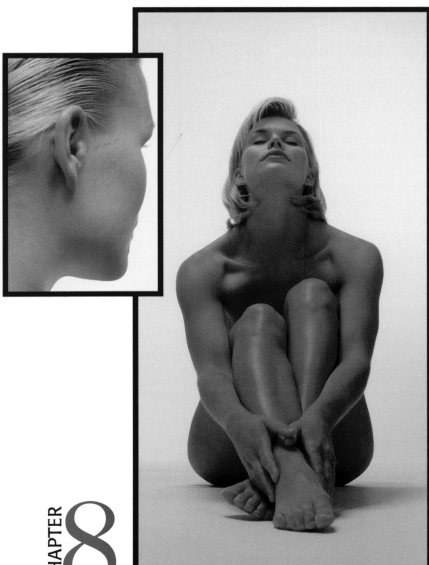

*Without
gravity we
would not
be here.
We would
be floating
somewhere
off in
outer space
and the way
we look would
probably be of
little concern.
Despite this
benefit, gravity
can also
be cruel.*

CHAPTER 8

Our agenda to uplift the skin includes:

▪ *facelift*
▪ *eyelid lift*
▪ *eyebrow lift*

FACELIFT

A popular misconception about facelifts (rhytidectomy) is that the signs of aging will be completely removed over the entire face. Instead, it is a procedure designed to improve the signs of aging, particularly redundant skin, in the lower half of the face, from the corners of the lips, over the cheeks to the neck level. It has no effect on the wrinkles around the eyes, the forehead or around the mouth.

Many people make the mistake of pulling the skin back tightly on the face so every wrinkle is removed in order to get an idea of what a facelift will do. The result is a mask-like appearance with the mouth and nose distorted. This is not what a facelift will do. A more accurate demonstration is to hold a mirror above the head and then look up into it. A tightening of the skin in the lower third of the face will be noted.

What signs of aging will a facelift correct?

A facelift is designed to correct three problems in the lower half of the face: poor muscle tone (which causes laxity in the neck and cheek regions); excess amounts of fat in the jowl, chin, and neck regions (sometimes referred to as a "turkey gobbler" deformity); and too much skin in the lower half of the face resulting in excessive wrinkling.

These problems are due to a combination of degenerative changes and the constant pull of gravity on the skin and muscles of the lower face. The occurrence and severity of the problems will vary from individual to individual depending on a person's inherited aging pattern and the amount of exposure they have had to sun, wind, and pollutants.

A facelift will not correct the vertical wrinkles that occur around the mouth due to muscle pull nor the crow's feet around the eyes. It is for this reason that many surgeons often combine a facelift with resurfacing. The facelift deals with the quantity of skin and the resurfacing with the quality of the skin.

Who is a candidate for facelift surgery?

If the lower half of the face has too much fat, poor muscle tone and lax skin as described above, then facelift surgery could correct these problems.

There is no "best" age for facelift surgery, although the average age tends to be approximately 50 to 55 years. As with other forms of cosmetic surgery, communication

Steps in Facial Surgery

Preparation for Surgery

1] A complete consultation with the surgeon to establish the goals for surgery as well as an understanding of the benefits and potential complications.

2] Written instructions may be given by physician.

3] Any blood test considered appropriate will be ordered.

4] Instructions are given not to take acetylsalicylic acid (aspirin) 2 weeks prior to and 1 week after surgery. This agent thins the blood and as a result may cause problems with increased bleeding and bruising during and after the procedure.

5] Smoking should be avoided 5 weeks prior to and 5 weeks after surgery as it inhibits healing due to blood vessel constriction.

6] If needed, pre-operative medication is provided and may include sedatives and antibiotics.

7] All makeup must be removed prior to surgery.

8] A photograph is taken prior to surgery. It is the best means of comparing post-operative results to the pre-operative condition.

9] Prior to anesthesia, the surgeon will plan the surgery by marking the skin with a pen while the patient is sitting. Hair in the area of the incision may be trimmed.

10] Facial surgery is usually performed on an outpatient basis. The patient returns home with a responsible adult who should remain with patient for a 12- to 24-hour period in case of unforeseen complications.

Post-operative Instruction

1] "DOs" and "DO NOTs" following surgery are given to the patient.

2] Bed rest is usually recommended for the remainder of the day.

3] The head should be slightly elevated when lying down so fluids drain away from the face. This helps to control swelling.

4] Painkillers and, in some circumstances, antibiotics are prescribed.

5] The dressing is usually removed by the surgeon the day after surgery.

6] A shower may be taken once dressings are removed and the hair can be gently shampooed. The incisions are dabbed dry after washing and left open to the air. Normally, no further dressings or ointments are applied.

7] Once the sutures are out and providing the wound or wounds are dry and healed, makeup may be used. It is best to avoid makeup directly on the incision for 2 weeks. Makeup to camouflage bruising may be applied after 1 week.

8] Sunscreens, sunglasses, and sun hats should always be worn after any facial surgery.

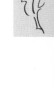

CHAPTER 8

Closure Lines for Facelifts

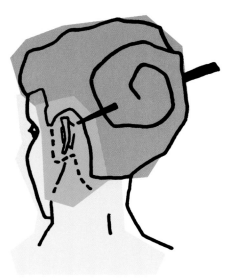

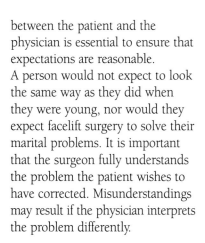

between the patient and the physician is essential to ensure that expectations are reasonable.

A person would not expect to look the same way as they did when they were young, nor would they expect facelift surgery to solve their marital problems. It is important that the surgeon fully understands the problem the patient wishes to have corrected. Misunderstandings may result if the physician interprets the problem differently.

What is involved in a facelift?

The table outlining the Steps in Facial Surgery apply to facelifts with a few unique differences. Facelift surgery is tailored to specific needs, but the basic steps are as follows:

■ A general or a local anesthetic may be administered. Intravenous sedation to relax the patient is often administered as well if local anesthetic is used.

■ Some of the hair above and behind the ear may have to be shaved if the incision is to be made in the hair-bearing skin of the scalp.

■ The incision, although always around the ear, will vary according to the problems to be corrected, the quality of the skin and the technique used. If an endoscope is used then the incision is not as long because the surgeon does not have to draw back the skin to see what he or she is doing. The endoscope allows the surgeon to view the

CHAPTER

8

area being treated through a lighted microscope housed within a narrow cannula (round rigid or flexible tube). This is accompanied by surgical tools and/or a laser fiber passed in or along the same cannula.

To minimize trauma during the procedure and to shorten the healing time endoscopic face lifts are becoming more and more popular. They also offers the advantage of an unmarked canvas (the facial skin) for additional procedures such as laser resurfacing and laser removal of blood vessels or pigment spots. As these procedures, especially laser resurfacing, can cause a lot of swelling an extensive, tight incision line may be compromised.

When excessive redundant skin needs to be removed and lax muscle needs to be redraped rather than simply repositioned and elevated, an open surgical approach rather than endoscopic technique is preferable.

- Once the incision is made, the skin over the cheek and neck areas is lifted away from the underlying fibrous tissue.

- If the neck muscle requires repair or if fat beneath the skin is to be removed, another incision is made under the chin in a natural crease.

- The supporting fibrous layer under the skin is then tightened.

- The excess fat is removed from the jowl, cheek, and chin regions by either cutting or liposuction techniques.

- The skin is pulled smoothly across the lower half of the face and the excess skin is removed.

- The incisions are closed.

What happens after facelift surgery?

After the surgery, a dressing resembling a nun's habit is put on. The patient is kept in the recovery room area for 1 to 2 hours until the intravenous medication wears off. They are then sent home with a responsible adult. No hospital stay is required in most instances as the entire procedure takes place on an outpatient basis. Bed rest, with the head elevated on pillows, is recommended for the rest of the day. After 24 to 48 hours, the surgeon will remove the dressing and check the incisions. Following this, the patient should gently wash the face, have a shower, and shampoo the hair. The sutures in front of the ear are removed 4 to 5 days later; at 10 days the remaining sutures are removed.

Will there be a scar?

After the skin is cut, an initially red scar will gradually fade to pink and finally become white. Esthetic surgeons cannot perform facelift surgery without scars. They are, however, trained to place

Facelift

BEFORE

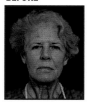

AFTER

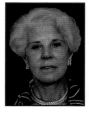

PHOTOS
COURTESY OF
CANADIAN SOCIETY
FOR AESTHETIC (COSMETIC)
PLASTIC SURGERY

CHAPTER 8

the scars in inconspicuous places so they will be barely noticeable when healing is complete.

Does facelift surgery hurt?

One of the greatest fears when considering a facelift is the pain. No pain will be felt during the surgery but, once the freezing wears off, there will be some discomfort along the incision line accompanied by a feeling of tightness in the neck region. Painkillers will usually be prescribed for the first 2 or 3 days of discomfort. Acetylsalicylic acid (aspirin) or similar products are not recommended because they tend to encourage bruising. A pulling, tender sensation behind the ear may be noticed, particularly when turning the head while sleeping. Once the sutures are removed or absorbed, this problem tends to subside.

Any severe pain in the area of the facelift may indicate a serious complication and the patient should contact their physician immediately.

Will there be any swelling and bruising?

An inevitable consequence of any surgical procedure is swelling and bruising although it tends to be less of a problem when lasers and endoscopic techniques are used. Swelling tends to be more prolonged in men. Swelling usually subsides in 10 to 14 days, although it may take as long as 6 weeks before the swelling completely disappears. Compresses may be helpful, but elevation of the head while lying down and time are the best healers.

When can normal activities be resumed?

We recommend that patients take at least 2 weeks off work, largely because of the cosmetic disability caused by the bruising and swelling. Any kind of normal activity that does not precipitate discomfort is allowed after 7 to 10 days. Strenuous physical activity and exercise should be avoided for approximately 4 to 6 weeks. It is best to use common sense: if it hurts, don't do it.

What are the most commonly asked questions?

The answers to the most commonly asked questions are as follows:

When can the hair be colored?

Three to 4 weeks after the surgery.

When can makeup be worn?

Two weeks after the surgery.

When can a depilatory or electrolysis be used to remove hair?

In 4 to 6 weeks, but, if the facelift is combined with a resurfacing technique, 12 weeks must pass.

How soon can a hair dryer be used?

Two weeks after surgery, although care should be taken to keep hot air away from the face for at least 4 weeks.

How soon can a facial be done?

Not until 6 weeks after surgery.

How long do the effects of the surgery last?

Facelift surgery does not prevent the face from aging. It simply sets the clock back, and this interval is usually maintained throughout life. For example, a 50-year-old who looks 55 may look 45 after a facelift. This 5 year advantage will be maintained throughout life. If at 60, the individual wants to look 55 again, another facelift will be required.

As many facelifts can be performed as desired; there are no restrictions. The surgery is personalized and addresses each specific problem as it occurs.

Are facelifts combined with other procedures?

Facelifts are frequently combined with laser resurfacing, chemical peels, brow lifts, and/or eyelid surgery. Each procedure improves an isolated area of the face. A combination of procedures to correct multiple areas of facial aging results in a better overall appearance than does a single procedure to correct an isolated problem.

What should men be aware of when considering facelifts?

Men undergo facelifts less often than do women and are generally less demanding in their expectations. Men have different hair patterns and a larger number of blood vessels because of facial hair. As a result of these differences, post-operative swelling tends to last longer in men, and the incidence of small blood clots is higher than in women. After surgery men will notice that their side burns are narrower because some of it will have been removed with the redundant skin.

What complications can occur?

■ **Scarring:** Unless there is a tendency to develop thick scars this will not be a serious complication. Scarring is an inevitable consequence of a surgical procedure where an incision has been made. Cosmetic surgeons try to hide scars but cannot prevent them.

Scars may form poorly because of an infection, an untreated blood clot, excess tension on the skin, or smoking after the surgery. If an unsatisfactory scar develops, a surgical scar revision procedure may need to be performed. If there is a tendency to form a thick scar even though it has healed well, further scar revision surgery will not be beneficial because a similar thick scar will form again with every surgical

CHAPTER 8

incision. This is an inherited healing characteristic. These scars can be flattened with cortisone injections and the redness reduced with a vascular removal laser. Lumpiness may be smoothed out by resurfacing the scar with a carbon dioxide laser.

Even if scarring is minimal, a skilled laser surgeon may improve the lines of closure by gently resurfacing these sites 6 to 10 weeks after surgery.

■ *Seroma:* Clear fluid may collect under the skin resulting in a seroma. These usually occur in the cheek area and feel like small firm lumps. In most cases, they reabsorb spontaneously in 4 to 6 weeks.

■ *Hematoma:* If blood collects under the skin, it is called a hematoma. The incidence of this is only 2% and tends to be more common in men than in women. Rapid swelling develops progressively on one side of the face with an increasing amount of pain and a feeling of tightness. If recognized early, it can be treated satisfactorily by removing the clot and stopping the bleeding. If the hematoma remains unrecognized, pressure under the skin might lead to skin loss and result in facial scarring. The increased bruising, swelling, and firmness that accompanies a hematoma will prolong recovery from surgery.

■ *Nerve Injury:* It is normal to have some loss of sensation in the face following the surgery. Sensation begins to return within 1 week and complete sensation is usually restored within 6 to 12 weeks. There is, however, a risk of injury to the nerve that supplies feeling to the ear. If this nerve is damaged, the sensation over the ear will be permanently decreased and there will be a small painful lump in the upper neck where the nerve was injured. Rarely will the nerve to the muscles that move the forehead and elevate the eyebrows be damaged. Injury to the muscle in the corners of the mouth is an uncommon occurrence, but if it does happen, the result will be a lopsided smile. The incidence of this is about 1 or 2 per thousand cases, and the majority of these recover spontaneously after 3 to 4 months.

■ *Infection and Skin Slough:* Infection is a rare complication in facelift surgery. As a precaution some esthetic surgeons will prescribe an antibiotic. If infection does occur and is extensive, some skin along the incision may die because the blood supply is interrupted. This can also occur because of excessive tension at the skin closure, a hematoma, or smoking after the operation. Eventually, the wound heals, but a thicker, wider scar will develop.

■ *Contour Irregularities:*

If small lumps or irregularities occur in the cheek area, they are commonly caused by a small hematoma or seroma.

They invariably subside with time (4 to 6 weeks) and do not require any specific treatment. Occasionally, irregularity in the neck region may occur if more fat has been removed from one side than from the other. This can be corrected by removing remaining fat with liposuction but only after a waiting period of 6 to 12 months. The waiting period is to ensure that the irregularity is not just asymmetrical swelling that resolves without surgery. Sometimes, the salivary gland beneath the jaw bone is quite prominent. If the gland was prominent before surgery but camouflaged by excess skin and fat, it will become more prominent after the surgery because the excess fat is removed and the skin is tightened.

What can be done if the surgery is unsatisfactory?

If the patient is dissatisfied with the facelift, and has not experienced any untoward complications he or she may have had unrealistic expectations in the first place. This may have occurred because the preliminary communication and consultation process between patient and physician did not clear up all the misconceptions about what facelift surgery could accomplish.

It can also happen that a complication following facelift surgery causes a less than satisfactory result. In these circumstances, revisional surgery could be performed to improve the disappointing results.

Who performs facelifts and how much do they cost?

A plastic surgeon trained in cosmetic facial surgery performs this surgery, in most cases, although other esthetic surgeons such as dermatologists and otolaryngologists may also be qualified. Therefore, it is up to the patient to check the credentials of the surgeon to ensure that he or she is properly trained to do the procedure. The cost of a facelift ranges from $2000 up to $8000. Other facial procedures done in combination with facelifts will affect these costs.

What are soft laser facelifts?

The use of soft or cool beam lasers has received some publicity and has been advertised by esthetic salons throughout North America and Europe. There is, however, no evidence to show that soft beam lasers permanently reduce wrinkles, as do surgical facelifts.

Medical lasers, such as the carbon dioxide laser, are surgical tools used to alter the skin by cutting or vaporizing. Soft lasers, which include gallium-arsenide and helium-neon, are not surgical lasers. They are

CHAPTER 8

light beams that enter the superficial layers of the skin causing some mild changes. Inflammation and subsequent edema (accumulation of fluid in the tissue) may actually make wrinkles temporarily less obvious because the fluid puffs them up. It is debatable whether the soft laser light enters the second layer of the skin to alter the collagen building block metabolism. More research is needed in this area. If it is determined that it does alter tissue it would be considered a medical instrument and cosmetic salons could no longer use them.

The soft laser light is often accompanied by an electrical impulse that contributes to further inflammation and accumulation of fluid in the tissue. It may also cause a temporary spasm of the muscles giving the appearance and sensation of tightness to the face, but this is only temporary.

Some soft lasers give the sensation of a single, brief, mildly uncomfortable pulse or wave of pulses that starts gently, reaches a peak, and then dies out. Others are completely painless. If the soft laser beam is accompanied by an electrical pulse, it is usually mildly uncomfortable. The treatments are generally given in 5 to 10 minute intervals for at least 20 sessions.

Are electric therapy facelifts beneficial?

As with soft laser facelifts, which are distinct from surgical facelifts that can be performed with a medical laser, electric therapy facelifts are controversial. Electric therapy is often used with soft lasers but may be used alone. A machine that delivers a very mild electric current is applied to the face causing some irritation and inflammation of the upper skin layers with subsequent edema. It may be applied on top of or into the skin using small needles. Insertion of needles is potentially dangerous and might lead to local infections, scarring, or transmission of such diseases as hepatitis or AIDS.

The current may cause temporary muscle spasms giving a sensation of tightness to the skin. It may also cause fluid shifts due to inflammation which puffs up fine wrinkles. This effect, however, is only temporary and lasts minutes, hours, or days, but certainly not longer. Anything causing excessive irritation or inflammation of the skin can cause damage. Most treatments involve 10 to 60 minute sessions every few days for several weeks and once a week thereafter.

There is considerable controversy over whether or not electric therapy is of any value whatsoever. Estheticians usually administer this therapy, but their training is variable and the types of equipment used differ widely. Risk is potentially small but certainly does exist, as it does with any device causing inflammation, irritation, and possible infection.

CHAPTER 8

Changes In The Eyelid With Age			
Childhood & adolescence	**20s to 40s**	**50s**	**60s to 70s**
Firm, wrinkle-free skin around eyes.	Fine wrinkles in eyelid.	Beginning of loose skin redundancy.	Redundant skin.
Firm muscle and eyelid tone.	Gradual development of crow's feet.	Prominent crow's feet.	Decrease in the tone of eyelids.
No fat.	Prominence of fat.	More fat.	Pronounced fat deposits.
No fluid.	Cyclical edema.	Lax muscle.	Lax muscle.
		Drooping eyebrow.	Drooping eyebrow.

Is acupuncture of any value in lessening wrinkles?

The insertion of small needles into the skin of the face will cause swelling and the puffing up of folds, creases, and wrinkles. This has the temporary effect of making the wrinkles appear less obvious. There is no long term benefit to acupuncture for the treatment of sagging, redundant skin and wrinkles.

EYELID LIFTS

The eyes play an important role in communication. They reflect emotions such as anger, fear, coyness, and happiness. Literary characters are frequently described in terms of their eyes. Yet, it is only the tissue around the eyes that is responsible for their dynamic expressions. The eyes themselves relay no message.

The skin around the eyes changes with age. It loses elasticity, becoming loose and redundant; the muscles around the eyes become slack; and excess fat in the pockets above and below the eyes become prominent. Cyclical edema or water in the tissue occurs with menstruation and certain sleep patterns.

The aging of the eyelids is largely determined by a genetic predisposition to the noted changes and by the amount of sun exposure received over time. The eyelids are also affected by gravity and muscle pull, such as habitual squinting. Allergies, cardiac problems, as well as thyroid and renal disorders can also be responsible for eyelid changes.

A surgical procedure called a blepharoplasty or eyelid plasty is commonly used to correct baggy eyelids. It is effective in removing excess skin and fat over the upper and lower eyelids and tightening up lax muscles around the eyes.

Who is a candidate for eyelid surgery?

Careful evaluation and medical examination is critical in ensuring a satisfactory result. A good candidate for eyelid surgery is a person with baggy eyelids due to excess fat, redundant skin, lax muscles around the eyes, and someone who has reasonable expectations.

Blepharoplasties will not be performed in the case of abnormal tear production (dry eyes), protruding eyes due to thyroid disease, nor other eye problems if surgery might endanger the eye or its vision.

Patients with high blood pressure, bleeding problems, glaucoma and diabetes mellitus are at risk for prolonged healing, bleeding during and after surgery and infection, therefore they are not good candidates for the surgery. Smokers are also not good candidates because their circulation is poor which results in a slow healing time and coughing after surgery may cause a blood vessel to burst which in turn could result in impaired vision.

Bags which form at the junction of the lower eyelids and upper part of the cheeks are medically referred to as malar bags. These bags are due to chronic swelling not muscle weakness or excessive fat accumulation and will not be improved by a blepharoplasty. Malar bags may be excised directly during eyelid surgery, but are best treated by laser resurfacing.

Eyelid Lifts

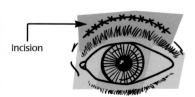

Incision

Single Approach to Upper Eyelid Lift

Upper eyelid suture line buried in upper eyelid crease

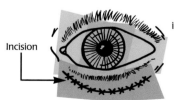

Incision

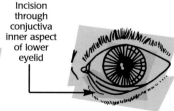

Incision through conjuctiva inner aspect of lower eyelid

Two Approaches to Lower Eyelid Lift

Lower eyelid incision line using external approach (sutures required)

Lower eyelid incision line (no sutures required)

CHAPTER 8

Blepharoplasty also cannot correct or alter deep, dark circles under the eyes, cyclical edema, allergies, crow's feet, and fine wrinkles around the eyes. Other types of intervention are required to deal with these problems. Medicated creams, collagen implants, laser resurfacing and chemical peels, all discussed previously, are alternatives for reducing wrinkles around the eyes.

Some surgeons divide the muscular ring around the eyes to help eliminate crow's feet while performing a blepharoplasty. This procedure, however, may weaken the eye muscles. A more promising alternative is the injection of botulinum toxin (Botox) into the muscles on the outside of the eyes to temporarily immobilize them so the crow's feet become less obvious. Another alternative is removal with laser resurfacing.

What takes place in a blepharoplasty?

The Steps in Facial Surgery chart also apply to blepharoplasties. When a facelift is combined with upper and lower eyelid surgery, the upper eyelids are corrected first. The surgeon will remove the appropriate amount of excess skin and fat, leaving symmetrical eyelids with inconspicuous incisions and well defined eyelid creases.

Upper Eyelid: The following are the steps taken to improve the upper eyelid (the procedure usually takes about one hour from start to finish):

- A surgical plan is drawn on the eyelids.

- A local anesthetic is administered. In most cases an intravenous sedation to relax the patient is used in conjunction with the local anesthetic.

- An incision is made with either a scalpel or a carbon dioxide laser. The CO_2 laser seals the blood vessels and nerve endings as it cuts so there is less bleeding during the procedure. If a scalpel is used bleeding is controlled with electrocautery.

- First the excess skin is removed which exposes the underlying muscle.

- A strip of muscle 5 to 8 millimeters (1/8 to 1/4 inches) wide is removed to create a deeper eyelid crease.

- Removal of the muscle exposes 2 fat pads. Excess fat is carefully removed.

- The incision is closed with absorbable sutures or if absorbable sutures are not used the stitches are removed in 3 to 5 days.

Lower Eyelid: There are two methods used to perform lower eyelid correction, an external incision technique or a transconjunctival technique:

CHAPTER 8

- In both cases a local anesthetic in combination with intravenous sedation is administered.

- The external technique involves the removal of excess fat, skin, and muscle, through an incision made in the skin just below the eyelashes. The eyelashes are never cut. When only excess fat, but no excess skin or muscle, is being removed an incision is usually made within the inner lining of the eyelid using the transconjunctival technique.

  A scalpel or the carbon dioxide laser may be used to make the incision. When the laser is used the procedure is much faster and so is the healing time because there is less bruising, swelling, and discomfort. For these reasons it is becoming a more popular choice for both surgeons and patients. Laser assisted blepharoplasties do, however, require more training and additional expenses for the cosmetic surgeon and hence it is not available in every center. Also many cosmetic surgeons still feel most comfortable with traditional scalpel surgery.

- Once the incision has been made below the lower eyelash using the external technique, a skin and muscle flap is created exposing three fat pads; the excess fat is carefully removed. A skin and muscle flap is not necessary when the incision is made in the inner lining of the conjunctiva because the fat pads are readily accessible. They are simply opened and the excess fat is removed. The surgeon is careful not to remove too much fat or the eye will have a sunken appearance.

- The transconjunctival technique is usually performed in concert with laser resurfacing to smooth out the texture of the skin and to remove the wrinkles around the eyes. It is for this reason that the excess skin and muscle do not need to be removed because the laser resurfacing causes the redundant skin to tighten. Sutures are not required when the transconjunctival technique is used, the incision is simply left to heal on its own.

- When the external technique is used, excess skin and muscle are removed. Care is taken not to remove too much skin or the sclera (the white part of the eye below the iris) will show . The incision is closed and sutures are removed or absorbed in 3 to 5 days.

Which technique is preferable, the transconjunctival or the external technique?

In most cases the transconjunctival technique using a CO_2 laser is preferable because:

- there is no visible incision, therefore no visible scar.

- there is no interference with the orbital septum (a membrane separating the outer tissue of the eye from the deeper tissue).
- there is less irritation and trauma to the eyelid because less traction is required during surgery.
- there is less interference with the shape of the lower lid.
- there is less bruising and swelling after the surgery.
- the incision inside the eyelid leaves the external eyelid free of trauma making it possible to resurface the skin with the laser at the same time that the blepharoplasty is performed.

Does the surgery hurt?

There is no pain during the surgery. As the freezing wears off, some discomfort will be felt which can easily be managed with painkillers. Acetylsalicylic acid (aspirin) products or similar agents should not be used as they encourage bleeding.

What will the eyes look like after surgery?

Some swelling and bruising will occur immediately after surgery, but it is unlikely the eyes will swell shut. It usually takes 10 to 14 days for swelling and bruising to disappear, thereafter normal activities can be resumed.

Eyelid surgery makes the eyes look brighter and wider. The puffiness from the excess fat will be gone as well as the redundant skin and bagginess. If the lower eyelid transconjunctival technique with the CO_2 laser is used in combination with laser resurfacing the wrinkles and texture changes around the eyes will also be improved. These problems are not addressed if the external technique is used.

Will there be a scar?

The incision for an upper lid blepharoplasty is placed in the crease of the eyelid so the scar will be inconspicuous when healed. Most eyelid scars fade rapidly after surgery and are quite faint in 6 weeks to 3 months. They may, however, take as long as 6 months to a year to fade, depending on how quickly the patient heals. The scar will not fade faster if a special diet is eaten or if creams such as vitamin E are applied. Makeup may be applied to camouflage the scar until it fades.

No visible scar occurs with a lower lid transconjunctival blepharoplasty because the incision is inside the eyelid. There is a scar just under the eyelashes of the lower lid when the external technique is used. In women this scar can be camouflaged with makeup, men however find it more difficult to manage and generally prefer the transconjunctival technique for this reason.

CHAPTER 8

Laser Eyelid Lift and Laser Resurfacing

BEFORE

AFTER

PHOTOS
COURTESY OF
DR. DON GROOT

When may makeup, glasses, and contact lenses be worn?

Makeup could be used to camouflage bruising 4 days after the surgery. Makeup, however, should not be applied to the actual scar until 10 days after surgery, and false eyelashes should not be used for 3 weeks.

Eyeglasses may be worn immediately after the surgery. Contact lenses should not be worn for at least 3 weeks to avoid pulling and stretching the incision.

Are there any restrictions on driving and flying?

Driving should be avoided for 2 or 3 days after the surgery. As to flying there is no restriction unless you are the pilot.

What is the ideal age for a blepharoplasty?

Cosmetic surgery, including that of the eyes, can be performed at any age. Anyone who feels young but looks old is a candidate for cosmetic surgery. The actual chronological age may be a consideration, only because younger tissue tends to recover better than older tissue does.

Can blepharoplasty be combined with other surgery?

Eyelid surgery is often performed in combination with other cosmetic procedures, such as laser resurfacing, facelifts, facial liposuction, and brow lifts.

How long do the effects of a blepharoplasty last?

The surgery does not stop the aging process, soft tissue around the eyes will continue to develop the signs of aging. It is, however, unlikely that a second full blepharoplasty will be needed. Usually, secondary procedures, such as lid tightening or laser resurfacing, are sufficient to correct minor imperfections around the eyes in the future.

What complications might occur after blepharoplasty?

■ *Scarring:* Scars normally fade to fine white lines and are only a problem in patients who are hereditarily predisposed to develop thick, raised scars. Even if a person is prone to scarring, it may nonetheless resolve itself over time. Minute amounts of cortisone sometimes are injected into the scar to flatten it and make it less obvious and one of the vascular lasers can remove persistent redness.

■ *Puffiness:* Occasionally, lid puffiness is prolonged due to a problem with the lymphatic vessels in the eyelids which, when functioning normally, reduce tissue fluid. This problem usually resolves itself over time.

■ *Scleral Show:* A problem that may occur with an external lower lid blepharoplasty is scleral show, where the whites of the eyes are exposed under the iris. This happens because the scar contracts as it heals, causing the edge of the lower eyelid to be pulled downward. This can occur even in the most carefully executed surgery. Scleral show can usually be resolved by upwardly massaging the lower lid on a regular basis over a period of time. If the problem does not resolve itself, then either too much skin was removed or the lower lid has poor tone. In the former case, a lid tightening procedure could be done. Any corrective surgery should be postponed a full year following the original surgery in order to ensure that healing is complete. If the lower eyelid is lax 6 months later, a wedge of tissue is removed from the outer third of the lower lid to tighten it.

Scleral show is unlikely with the transconjunctival lower eyelid lift because no skin is removed with this technique. Texture changes and loose skin are treated with laser resurfacing.

■ *Lack of symmetry:* If one eyelid looks different from the other after surgery, it is usually due to a difference in the amount of scarring and swelling in each lid. In most cases, this is resolved over time, as the scar heals and the swelling subsides. If the problem persists, either the eyelids were different before the operation and the surgeon did not take this into account, or some variation in the surgery occurred from one eyelid to the other. This is why eyes are always photographed prior to surgery.

■ *Eyelid Lag:* An inability to close the eyelids completely is a temporary complication which resolves as the swelling settles and the scar fades. It may be necessary to protect the cornea from drying out until the problem is resolved.

■ *Numbness:* Numbness around the eyes may occur, but this is usually temporary and slowly resolves over a few months.

■ *Hematoma:* Although extremely rare, excessive bleeding may put pressure on the eye which may result in altered vision or blindness.

What results cause dissatisfaction?

In some cases there may be excess skin remaining in the eyelids. It is usually seen as a drooping eyebrow. A brow lift, rather than further surgery to the eyelid, will correct this problem .

If the lower lids continue to sag, it may be due to malar bags, which are best treated with laser resurfacing.

Eyelid surgery will not remove crow's feet. Laser resurfacing is the best treatment alternative for crow's

CHAPTER 8

feet. However, if a person prefers not to go through the post surgical recovery time required for laser resurfacing, collagen injections may be a reasonable alternative.

Noticeable contour irregularities may be due to bulges that occur when there has not been enough fat removed from the fat pads. This is easily corrected by removing more fat. At the other extreme, the eye may look hollowed out or sunken if too much fat has been removed.

Eyelid surgery will not remove dark circles under the eye. In fact, it may worsen the problem because, with removal of fat, the resulting concavity will give an illusion of even darker circles. A daily application of bleaching agents such as hydroquinone or kojic acid is helpful in reducing dark circles under the eyes if they are due to pigment changes in the skin and not the underlying vasculature showing through the thin transparent skin of the lower eyelid. It may also be possible to resolve the problem using a pigment removal laser such as the Q-switched ruby, Alexandrite, or Nd:Yag systems, although this is not always effective.

Prolonged discoloration following extensive bruising may occur but is usually resolved within a few weeks. In unusual cases, it may take 1 to 2 years to disappear, but bruises are rarely permanent.

Can eyelid surgery affect vision?

The surgeon is always very careful when working in the area of the eye, since there is a danger that the eye itself could be harmed.

Though rarely a problem, excess swelling and large hematomas could cause enough pressure around the eye to affect a person's sight and in the worst case scenario may cause blindness. For this reason, the physician will monitor vision carefully.

What are the alternatives to eyelid surgery?

In the early stages of eyelid drooping, resurfacing with the CO_2 laser may be adequate to tighten the skin around the eyes so that eyelid surgery can be postponed for a number of years.

Other alternative approaches for improving the eye area are either hazardous or ineffective. Injecting silicone implants into the eyelids to fill the skin out is medically unsound. Steroid injections into the fat pads in order to shrink the fat have proven to be unsuccessful.

Who performs blepharoplasties and what is the cost?

Plastic surgeons, dermatologists, and ophthalmologists specializing in esthetic facial surgery may perform blepharoplasties. As with other forms of cosmetic surgery, it is up to the patient to ensure that the esthetic surgeon is qualified to perform the procedure.

The cost varies with the surgeon's geographic location, the skill and experience of the surgeon, and the technique used. A bilateral upper and lower blepharoplasty may cost between $1,500 and $5,000.

BROW LIFT

Ideally, a woman's eyebrows should arch on or slightly above the upper orbital rims (upper rim of the bone over the eye) and a man's should arch along the rims. If the eyebrows are displaced downward, the face may portray certain stereotype expressions. For example, downward displacement of the inner portion of the eyebrows often depicts an expression of ill will; downward displacement of the middle portion of the eyebrows may depict an expression of sadness; and overall downward displacement of the eyebrows suggests fatigue. Similarly, forehead wrinkles relay certain facial expressions. Deep vertical lines between the eyebrows (in the glabellar region) give the unintentional impression of anger, annoyance, or a scowl, whereas a heavily lined forehead may give a tired and worried expression.

People with low set eyelids may have been born with them or they may be due to gravitational pull. More commonly, though, they are a manifestation of biological aging, which is determined by hereditary factors, and time (chronological aging). Gravitational pull on the skin of the forehead aggravates the problem.

Brow lift surgery improves the face dramatically by creating a brighter, softer, fresher appearance. It lifts heavy eyebrows away from the eyes and smooths out vertical lines between the eyebrows and transverse lines across the forehead.

Careful assessment by the surgeon is critical to ensure a satisfactory cosmetic result. Frequently, droopy eyebrows and excess eyelid skin are a combined problem. If this is the case, simply removing some eyelid skin will not correct the problem. In fact, it may worsen it by creating a shortage of skin in the upper lid causing the brow to be pulled down further.

If both a brow lift and blepharoplasty are found to be necessary, it is important to place the eyebrow in its correct position by performing the brow lift surgery first. In this way, less upper eyelid skin is removed during the blepharoplasty, thus preventing any problems with eyelid closure.

Brow lift surgery for forehead wrinkles is particularly effective in correcting droopy eyebrows as well. If, however, droopy eyebrows are not the problem, other options may be considered, including laser resurfacing, collagen implants or muscle relaxants such as Botox.

A "sinking" nose and excess nasal skin can be corrected with a brow lift, as an alternative to a rhinoplasty (nose job). Asymmetrical eyebrows, where one side sits higher than the other, may be improved by lifting the brow on the droopy side.

What is involved in a brow lift?

The basic steps for brow lift surgery are the same as those outlined in the table on the Steps for Facial Surgery. Three surgical techniques are used, each having distinct advantages and disadvantages:

■ The coronal technique is an incision made either in the scalp or at the junction of the scalp hair and forehead.

■ The mid-forehead technique involves an incision made within the natural creases of the mid-forehead.

■ The direct technique locates the incision just within the hairline of the upper part of the eyebrow.

The coronal technique is the most popular because the incision is hidden by the hair. By partially removing some of the muscle as well as the redundant skin, furrows and wrinkles on the forehead can be smoothed out at the same time the brows are lifted.

The most up-to-date method of performing the coronal technique utilizes a laser and an endoscope. An endoscope is a small round tube or cannula through which a light, a microscope and the fiber optics of the laser are passed. With conventional scalpel surgery the

incision is made from ear to ear across the top of the forehead just within the hair line. The incision is much smaller with the laser and endoscopic technique; 1 to 2 centimeters if reduction of the forehead and glabellar (between the eyebrows) wrinkles is the goal and a bit longer if a brow lift is also being performed. An improved visual field is possible because the laser seals off the blood vessels. The endoscope allows the surgeon to work under the skin without having to pull the entire skin flap away from the forehead.

The mid-forehead technique reduces wrinkling on the forehead and lifts droopy eyebrows, however, the disadvantage is that the scar is visible on the forehead.

The direct method does not reduce the wrinkles on the forehead; it is strictly a technique for lifting the brows. The surgeon can more accurately position the brow with this method, a particularly important consideration when the brows are asymmetrical.

Will there be a scar?

The incision with the conventional coronal technique heals with a cosmetically acceptable, fine white scar which is normally camouflaged within the hair. The scar, however, will be more obvious in balding men and women with diffuse hair loss. At first the scar may feel bumpy and irregular but becomes smooth and flat within 6 months.

The incisions with the laser and endoscopic coronal technique are very small and therefore easier to camouflage. In women the incision is usually placed behind the hairline in the middle of the scalp. In men and some women who show signs of male pattern hair loss 2 incisions are made on either side of the head, behind the hair line just above the ears. In this manner the scar is much less obvious in these individuals because hair loss normally takes place on top of the head.

Scars from incisions made on the forehead are visible. They are generally pink for 6 months, then gradually fade to a fine white line. The scars from the direct technique follow the same healing pattern but are somewhat camouflaged by the hair of the eyebrows.

Troublesome scars can be treated with a combination of injections and laser therapy. Cortisone injections will flatten raised scars, the vascular removal lasers will eliminate excess redness, and resurfacing with the carbon dioxide laser can even out the lumps and bumps of a scar to improve the texture.

How long does brow lift surgery take and does it hurt?

The length of surgery varies with the technique being used and the extent of the correction.

The actual surgery is painless because a local anesthetic is used to numb the area prior to the procedure. After the freezing wears off, some discomfort may be felt along the incision. A temporary headache and tightness of the forehead and scalp may also be experienced. Oral painkillers are all that is needed to relieve this discomfort, but no acetylsalicylic acid (aspirin) products should be used.

When can normal activities be resumed?

With conventional surgery swelling and bruising will last approximately 7 to 10 days, whereas with the laser and endoscopic method, the recovery period is only 3 to 4 days. Most people do not feel presentable in public until the initial stages of swelling and bruising have passed. Elevation of the head is recommended until the swelling has subsided. When this occurs any normal activity which does not precipitate discomfort is allowed.

How will surgery affect the face?

A conventional coronal brow lift will raise the hairline and a hairstyle change may be recommended if the change is quite dramatic. This is not as significant a problem when the laser and endoscopic technique is used.

A softer, brighter, more alert and youthful look will be noticed after the procedure. The appearance of the upper eyelids is also improved and the eyes will look wider. It is not uncommon to receive compliments on a well-rested happy look after brow lift surgery.

How long does the result last?

Brow lift surgery does not prevent aging. Lines of expression over the forehead and between the eyebrows will still be present, although to a much lesser extent. With time, they become more pronounced but the youthful effect created by the surgery remains for a prolonged period of time.

What are the possible complications of a brow lift?

■ **Prolonged Redness of the Scar:**
This is unusual and of significance only in cases where the incision has been made in the forehead. The scar may also be tender and lumpy. Eventually this subsides but it may take 1 to 2 years. The vascular lasers (pulsed dye or variable pulse width) can be used to remove the redness. Injections of cortisone and resurfacing with the carbon dioxide laser can smooth out raised and uneven scar tissue. Medications and ointments are not effective in speeding up the healing process. Makeup can be used to camouflage a scar until it has healed.

■ **Balding:** Men, and less so women, with male-pattern hair loss or a strong family history of balding are cautioned about scarring. As balding progresses, a scalp scar will become more and more apparent because it is no longer hidden within the hair. A scalp incision often accelerates hair loss because of the tension of the scar and the subsequent interruption of the blood supply to the scalp. Other causes of hair loss in the region of the scar are infection and hematoma, both of which are rare. This is much less of a problem with the laser and endoscopic technique.

■ **Loss of Sensation:**
Often, a transient loss of sensation over the forehead and scalp to the crown of the head is felt. Feeling returns to the forehead within 4 to 6 weeks and to the scalp after 6 to 9 months. The smaller incisions used with the laser and endoscopic technique significantly reduce the occurrence of this complication.

■ **Overcorrection:** If too much skin is removed, the face may look surprised or startled. With time, gravity's effect will improve this result. Overcorrection is often accompanied by too much tension at the scalp incision. This may cause poor healing, a wide scar, and hair loss.

CHAPTER

8

■ **Itching:** This may be troublesome, especially in the scalp area behind the incision. Fortunately this eventually subsides as the incision heals.

■ **Muscle Weakness:** Muscle weakness is usually a temporary condition which gradually disappears. A positive aspect of this is that the forehead furrows markedly diminish with relaxed muscles.

What are the alternatives to brow lift surgery?

Collagen implants or muscle relaxants are alternatives to brow lift surgery for deep furrows on the forehead. Droopy eyebrows, however, require some form of surgery. Laser resurfacing of the forehead may tighten the skin above the brow enough to give droopy eyebrows a bit of a lift. If the eyebrows are really heavy then a brow lift is the only option available.

Camouflage is another alternative to consider if drooping eyebrows are the problem. The outside half of the eyebrows can be plucked and another pencilled in higher up to create a more alert appearance and to eliminate the expression of fatigue. The effect does not match that of the brow lift, but is an alternative which avoids surgery.

Who performs brow lifts and what do they cost?

Plastic surgeons usually perform brow lift surgery, although dermatologists, ophthalmologists and other esthetic surgeons with special training in facial surgery, may also use this procedure. It is up to the patient to ensure that the surgeon is properly qualified.

The average price range for brow lift surgery is $1,000 to $3,000.

CHAPTER 8

Facial *Harmony*

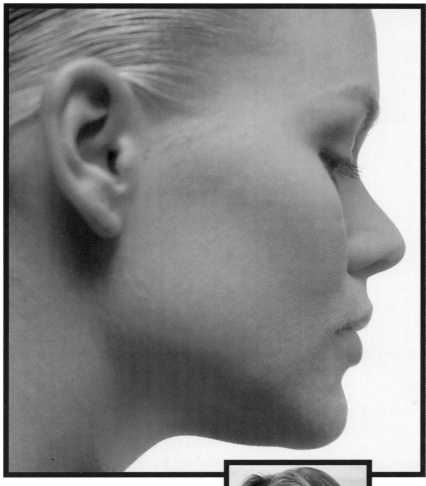

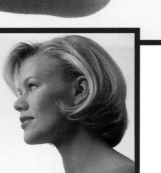

THE SHAPE OF THE FACE

As with most things in life, a sense of balance is important to your face. Most people are not blessed with perfectly proportioned facial features, but seem to be perfectly satisfied with what nature has given them.

9
CHAPTER

In gambling, you play the cards you're dealt, but that's not always necessary with those cards nature has dealt.

Our agenda for harmonious facial features includes:

- *nose*
- *chin*
- *cheeks*
- *jowls and neck*

Eleanor had lived most of her young adult life as a recluse. Her problems had begun in junior high school when her classmates had teased her about her nose. Such comments as "You'll never get lost with a nose like that to guide you" were common, and she frequently ran home in tears. Hating the way she looked, Eleanor avoided social contact. Studious behavior in university protected her from having to interact with her peers. Despite her level of education, Eleanor sought work which would minimize her contact with others.

Turning 30 was Eleanor's wake up call. Where had her youth gone, and what was she going to do with the rest of her life? She couldn't spend it hiding away. An article on cosmetic surgery in a woman's magazine had caught her interest. Was it possible a cosmetic surgeon could help her? It was worth a try. The surgeon was empathetic and, to Eleanor's surprise, had helped many people with similar

problems. A profiloplasty was recommended, and Eleanor underwent surgery to reduce the size of her nose, augment her chin, and remove some fat from her cheeks in order to emphasize her naturally high cheek bones. The transition in Eleanor's appearance mirrored the transition in her outlook on life. In her mind she was no longer an ugly duckling and her self-confidence and self-esteem soared.

The symmetry and shape of our face whether we are male or female determine to a large extent our attraction to the opposite sex. Studies have shown that it is the degree to which the right and left sides of our faces match that determine how attractive our faces appear to others.

The shape of the face is determined by bone and cartilage structures, the distribution of muscle and fat, and the way the skin drapes over bones and subcutaneous tissue. These factors in turn are determined by genetic makeup and racial origin.

Despite the mythical nature of common assumptions, personality traits and attractiveness are attributed to certain structural features. Examples: high cheek bones are associated with sophisticated beauty; a small, slightly turned-up nose is associated with youth and innocence; a square jaw is suggestive of strength; and a recessed chin gives the impression of weakness.

CHAPTER

Although misleading, the shape of the face may inadvertently and subliminally affect the assumptions made when people meet for the first time. These culturally based attitudes are often reinforced by cartoonists and comedians.

Men are routinely attracted to women with high arched eyebrows, wide open eyes, pronounced cheekbones, full lips, and shorter jaw lines. These traits apparently trigger a male's animal instinct for approachability and fertility. Women on the other hand look for large eyes, prominent cheekbones, a strong jaw line and chin, and a big smile. They also prefer a clean shaven to a bearded face. These traits would suggest on first impression that the male has the requisite requirements to fertilize and protect the nest in a nonaggressive manner.

If you look at your face in profile, you will see certain structural proportions that dictate the norms of facial harmony. If you draw a vertical line connecting the forehead, lower lip, and chin, they should all protrude to the same extent. The angle of the nose from the lip, according to Western standards, should be within 90 to 110 degrees. Inevitably, most people are not proportionally perfect, but are within an acceptable range.

Modern medicine allows alteration of some disproportionate features of the face. In cases like Eleanor's, the change may be dramatic, yet for others a subtle change, such as higher cheek bones, may be all that is desired.

A profiloplasty is a common medical term for the alteration of the structural proportions that determine a person's profile. One or several procedures may be recommended to improve the profile. Proportion and balance are the keys to success of any procedure that seeks to change the structure of the face and, more often than not, a combination of procedures may be necessary to obtain the desired result. An esthetic surgeon will be able to advise you as to your best approach.

NOSE

Today's occidental concept of a beautiful nose emphasizes angularity. This type of nose has a straight nasal bridge separated from the forehead by a shallow groove. The width of the nasal bridge is uniform along its entire length. A pleasing nasal tip is narrow and stands out from the straight nasal bridge. The nostrils are thin and gently drop to a narrow nasal base. The angle of the nose from the tip is usually 90 to 100 degrees. The impression of angularity is further enhanced by thin nasal skin. The goal of surgery, then, is to create an esthetically pleasing nose with nasal tip projection and angularity in mind, while maintaining facial harmony and balance.

9
CHAPTER

BEFORE

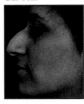

AFTER

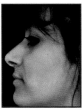

PHOTOS
COURTESY OF
CANADIAN SOCIETY
FOR AESTHETIC
(COSMETIC)
PLASTIC SURGERY

Rhinoplasty

The face is the most visible part of the body, but the nose is its most prominent feature. It is not surprising therefore that nasal surgery is one of the most common procedures in North America. Rhinoplasty is the term used for nasal surgery.

The first rhinoplasties were performed to reduce large noses. Today, similar procedures are followed to reduce excess amounts of bone, cartilage, and fat in the nose in order to make it more esthetically pleasing. Making the nose larger (augmentation rhinoplasty) to achieve a desired esthetic result has also gained in popularity. This may involve adding cartilage from the nasal septum or from the ear to the bridge and tip of the nose. Silastic (silicone) implants are also frequently used. An augmentation rhinoplasty can help those who are unhappy with an unsuccessful reduction rhinoplasty.

The surgeon is frequently asked to create the same nose as a model's in a glossy magazine. It is not possible to surgically duplicate a nose. This is because anatomic characteristics differ from one person's nose to another's.

Before surgery, the physician will ask the patient about any difficulty with nasal obstruction. Intranasal examination may reveal some obstruction to the nasal

airway which could be corrected simultaneously.

In addition, the surgeon assesses facial balance, including the neck, chin, upper lip, forehead, cheek-bone areas, and glabella (the area between the eyebrows). A surgical plan based on the esthetic goals is then established and thoroughly discussed with the patient.

If the patient is over 50, and wishes to undergo a reduction rhinoplasty, he or she should be aware that there may be an excess amount of nasal skin after the surgery. Due to the loss of elasticity and resiliency experienced with age, the skin does not shrink to the new shape of the nose. Usually this problem is anticipated by the surgeon and is corrected by removing the excess skin or, in some cases, by lifting the brow.

What does a rhinoplasty involve?

The Steps in Facial Surgery in Chapter 8 apply to a rhinoplasty. Most esthetic rhinoplasties are performed under local anesthesia with intravenous sedation, although general anesthetics are used in some situations.

The surgery involves a series of incisions within the nose and occasionally across its base. These incisions enable the surgeon to reach the cartilage, bone, and fat of the nose. Depending on the goal, these tissue components will be modified to produce an esthetically pleasing result. The bone of the nose is often broken as part of the surgery, and this accounts for most of the bruising and swelling around the eyes following the procedure. The incisions are closed with sutures that are absorbed within 7 to 10 days. The nose is often packed with a small amount of vaseline gauze which is removed the following day. Tape or a plaster-of-paris cast is applied to the nose, and this is removed 7 to 10 days following the surgery.

After the intravenous sedation has worn off (within 1 to 2 hours), the patient is sent home with a responsible adult to rest quietly with the head elevated.
The following day the packing is removed, either by the patient or the surgeon.

Will the surgery hurt?

After the freezing wears off some discomfort is felt in the nasal area for 1 to 2 hours but quickly subsides with oral painkillers (no aspirin). Headaches following the surgery are common but are also managed with painkillers.
It is unusual to feel significant discomfort in the nasal area the day following the surgery. After the cast is removed, the nose is tender to the touch for approximately 3 months.

Some discomfort may be experienced when the head is bent forward because of pressure due to swelling. As swelling subsides, so will the discomfort.

Will there be any swelling and bruising?

Some swelling and bruising occurs, particularly if the nose has been fractured. Occasionally, bleeding occurs under the clear lining over the eyes, making them red and blotchy. This is not harmful, other than looking quite unsightly for about 3 weeks. Most of the bruising and swelling subsides within 7 to 10 days.

Will there be a scar?

Most of the incisions are inside the nose and are not visible. Occasionally, a small scar may be seen at the base of the nose if the nostrils were narrowed or an external nasal approach was used.

How long will it take to heal?

Since the skin over the upper section of the nose is thinner than on the lower section, each section heals at a different rate. Within 6 weeks, the swelling subsides in the upper portion of the nose. Due to the thickness of the skin over the nasal tip, however, it takes a longer period of time for the swelling in the lower part of the nose to subside. The tip of the nose feels firm and fibrous in the weeks following surgery. Gradually, the tip of the nose becomes more pliable. Complete healing of the tip of the

CHAPTER 9

nose usually takes 6 to 9 months, but in some cases might take as long as one year.

Can the surgery be redone?

Surgery may be performed again if the original results are disappointing. A one year healing period must pass before further surgery to ensure that all scars within the nose have healed and that no further changes will take place. A follow-up appointment is made within one year to confirm that esthetic goals have been achieved. A second photograph is usually taken at this time.

What are the possible complications of rhinoplasty?

Complications are uncommon. An unsatisfactory esthetic appearance is the usual concern. Swelling, bruising, and a firm fibrotic feel to the nose are normal consequences of rhinoplasty. Occasionally, the nasal skin will be rosy following surgery.

Small dilated veins sometimes remain after the bruising and swelling subside. These can be removed with one of the vascular removal lasers. Infections are rare, but are readily treated with antibiotics.

When can makeup, glasses, and contact lenses be worn?

Glasses sit quite comfortably on top of the nasal cast. Once the cast is removed it is preferable to wear contact lenses to avoid any pressure that glasses may exert on the recently fractured nose until the bones have healed completely. Makeup may be worn once the cast is removed.

When can normal activities be resumed?

Ordinarily, normal activities may be resumed within 1 to 2 weeks. Driving can be resumed the following day, provided there is no excessive swelling about the eyes that restricts vision. If an obstruction inside the nose was corrected at the time of surgery, flying should be avoided for 7 to 10 days because pressure changes might cause the nose to bleed.

Who performs rhinoplasties and what is the cost?

Plastic surgeons and otolaryngologists perform rhinoplasties at a cost of $1,500 to $6,000.

CHIN

When the chin is out of proportion with the rest of the face it may detract from the attractiveness of the other features. In the extreme, a jaw that is too large or small affects dental occlusion and requires the attention of orthodontists and oral surgeons. Orthognathic surgery to correct more serious problems with the jaw is discussed in the chapter on the teeth.

Even though the dental occlusion is normal, the chin may be out of balance with the rest of the face. It may be recessed or too small, too pointed or crooked, too short or long, or it may protrude too much. The disproportionate chin may be corrected in two ways (if no dental malocclusion exists): a chin implant can be inserted or the bone of the jaw can be adjusted.

Chin Implants

Chin implants are usually made of a silastic (silicone) material and are available in two forms: as a gel within a bag, or as a solid block which is either preformed or contoured to each individual need. Acrylic implants may also be used.

Implant surgery usually takes approximately 30 minutes, and is performed under a local anesthetic. After rinsing the mouth with an antiseptic mouthwash, an incision is made in the depression between the lower lip and the external gums of the lower teeth. A pocket is then created between the lining of the bone and the muscle and fat covering the chin. The size of the pocket is determined by the structure of the face and the esthetic goals. An implant to fit the pocket is then put in place and the incision is closed. The advantage to this procedure is that there is no external scar.

In the past, the incision was made in the natural crease under the chin. Although the scar was somewhat hidden in the crease, it was still visible. This is why entering through the mouth is now preferred. Once the procedure is complete, a light pressure dressing is applied to control swelling and bruising. The dressing is removed within 2 days.

For comfort, a soft diet is recommended until the dressings are removed. Hot foods should also be avoided because the area tends to be numb for some time after the surgery and there is a risk of scalding the lower lip.

Will there be any pain after surgery?

Only mild discomfort is felt for the first few days after surgery because of the pressure the implant and swelling exert in the area of the chin. As the swelling subsides, so does the discomfort.

The incision within the mouth is irritating for the first few days, just as with any sore in that area. A mild painkiller helps to minimize the discomfort until the swelling subsides, usually within 7 to 10 days.

When can normal activities be resumed?

Normal activities can be resumed within 2 days, once the pressure dressing has been removed.

CHAPTER 9

Are there any potential complications?

The most common complication is a loss of sensation in the lower lip and chin region. Due to swelling, pressure is exerted on the nerve supply to the area. This loss of sensation is usually temporary and will return to normal in several weeks.

Other complications with this procedure are rare but may include:

- Extrusion or expulsion of the implant, usually as a result of infection or a pocket that is too tight.

- Erosion of the jawbone at the site of the implant occurs if the implant is placed directly on the bone rather than on the lining of the bone. If the implant is placed too high, erosion of the bone above the implant may cause damage to the dental roots.

- A poorly positioned implant will create an unsatisfactory cosmetic result.

Implants may easily be replaced or removed through the original incision in the event of any of these complications or if the results are disappointing.

Can chin implants be combined with other procedures?

A chin implant is often combined with a rhinoplasty. Liposuction is also commonly done in conjunction with chin implants; fat is sucked from jowls, and under the chin, the cheeks, and the neck. This contouring provides the finishing touch to the proportional changes that are accomplished with rhinoplasty and chin implants.

Who inserts chin implants and what do they cost?

Plastic surgeons, otolaryngologists, and oral surgeons trained in cosmetic surgery of the face are specialists who would perform this procedure. The cost of the procedure varies from $500 to $2,000.

Jawbone Adjustment

The second and less common procedure used to correct a disproportionate chin is an adjustment to the jawbone. Unlike the chin implant, which augments the chin region with foreign material, an adjustment to the jawbone utilizes the patient's own bone tissue.

Although the procedure is done on an outpatient basis, a general anesthetic is usually administered. As with chin implants, the incision is made within the mouth after the mouth has been rinsed with an antiseptic mouthwash.

To adjust the jawbone, it must be released from the rest of the jawbone. This is accomplished by cutting the bone horizontally just under the roots of the lower teeth, then vertically down at the eyeteeth.

Once separated, the chin may be shortened by removing some of the bone, lengthened by pulling the bone forward, tilted up to shorten the vertical dimension of the face, or tilted down to lengthen the vertical dimension of the face. A permanent stainless steel wire is used to fix the bone into its new position. Once the bone has been wired into place, the incision within the mouth is closed. There is no visible scar after the procedure.

A pressure dressing is applied around the chin to control subsequent swelling and bruising. The dressing is removed after 1 to 2 days. As with implants, a soft diet is recommended until the dressings are removed. Hot foods should also be avoided.

Will there be pain after surgery?

Moderate discomfort is experienced during the first few days after the surgery due to the severed bone and the pressure exerted in the chin area by swelling. As the swelling subsides, so does the discomfort. Unlike a chin implant, where mild discomfort is experienced for 1 or 2 days, a jawbone adjustment may cause discomfort for a couple of weeks or more. As is the case with chin implants, the incision within the mouth will be irritating for the first few days. Pain medication is generally recommended as an effective means of controlling discomfort. The swelling

and bruising will be greater than that experienced with a chin implant and generally subsides within 10 days.

Will there be a scar?

Yes, but the scar is in the mouth and cannot be seen.

When can normal activities be resumed?

Most patients are able to return to their normal routine after a period of 3 to 4 days.

What are the potential complications?

A temporary loss of sensation to the lower lip and chin region caused by pressure on the nerve supply due to swelling may occur. It often takes several weeks for sensation to return to normal.

Another complication is the possibility of an infection which may occur because the bone has been temporarily detached from its blood supply.

Can chin surgery be combined with other surgery?

As with chin implants, bone adjustments are often combined with rhinoplasties and liposuction to the jowls, under the chin, the cheeks, and the neck. This total approach often achieves the best cosmetic result.

CHAPTER

What are the advantages and disadvantages of a jawbone adjustment over a chin implant?

A jawbone adjustment eliminates the risk of erosion of the bone, damage to the teeth, and extrusion or expulsion of the implant. It also uses the patient's own tissue rather than a foreign substance, which leaves the chin with a more natural feel when it is touched.

The disadvantage of a jawbone adjustment is that it is a more extensive procedure and requires a general anesthetic with its inherent risks. Other risks are loss of sensation to the lower lip for a longer period of time and potential infection. This procedure also has more restrictions on the size to which the chin may be enlarged.

Who performs chin surgery and what does it cost?

Plastic surgeons, otolaryngologists, and oral surgeons trained in esthetic surgery of the face are specialists who perform this surgical procedure.

The range in cost is $2,000 to $5,000.

CHEEKS

High cheek bones are considered to be a feature of beauty in North American society. Although cheek implantation is not a common cosmetic procedure, it alters the structure of the face by enlarging and raising the cheekbone area as well as widening the face. Reshaping the skin over the implant also makes the wrinkles under the eyes less obvious.

Cheek implants are frequently combined with other types of cosmetic surgery: rhinoplasties, facelifts, liposuction, and chin implants.

Cheek Implants

Materials used for cheek implants include silastic bags, silastic blocks (either preformed or contoured to the exact needs of the individual), acrylic, and bone. Bone is used more in extensive reconstructive surgery than in cosmetic enhancement surgery.

An incision is made either just under the lower eyelashes or through the mouth along the upper portion of the gums. A pocket is created between the cheekbone lining and the subcutaneous tissue. As with chin implants, the size of the pocket determines the size of the implant. In turn, the size of the pocket is determined by facial structure and esthetic goals.

Once the implant is in place, the incision is closed and a pressure dressing is usually applied over the implant to control swelling and bruising. The dressing is removed after one to two days, although swelling and bruising take about 2 weeks to subside.

9
CHAPTER

YOUNG AS YOU LOOK

Do the cheeks hurt after surgery?

Mild discomfort is felt initially due to swelling and pressure from the implant. As the swelling subsides so does the discomfort. Mild painkillers are effective for controlling discomfort.

What are the possible complications with this procedure?

As with chin implants, sensation over the cheeks may temporarily be affected due to pressure on the nerves supplying the area. Normal sensation will usually return once the swelling has subsided. It is extremely rare that sensation in the area is permanently altered.

Extrusion or expulsion of the implant is also a rare occurrence and is associated with a pocket that is too small, or an unexpected infection.

If the implant is poorly positioned, it can be adjusted or replaced through the original incision.

What do cheek implants cost and who performs the surgery?

The price ranges from $1,500 to $3,000. Plastic surgeons and oral surgeons perform cheek implant surgery.

JOWLS AND NECK

As we age the fat in our face becomes redistributed. Fat may gather in the lower portion of the face in pouches at the base of the cheeks known as jowls or under the chin. The chin may look as if it is lost or redundant.

Tumescent liposuction can significantly improve a person's looks when the fat has begun to gather in the lower portion of the face. If the accumulation of fat is accompanied by a loss of elasticity in the skin then a combination of liposuction and a face lift must be considered.

What is involved in tumescent liposuction of the jowls and neck?

Tumescent liposuction has been discussed in depth in Chapter 15 but there are some unique characteristics of liposuction to the face.

■ The incision sites are anesthetized.

■ Tiny incisions for tumescent liposuction of the jowls are made on either side of the mouth in the crease between the nose and the corners of the lips as well as along the under portion of the jaw line.

■ Tiny incisions for tumescent liposuction of the chin are placed along the under portion of the

CHAPTER

jaw line and centrally along the vertical line of the throat.

- A solution of saline, lidocaine, epinephrine, cortisone and bicarbonate is injected into the subcutaneous fat to be removed. The saline increases the volume of the fat making it easier to remove and allows a natural and attractive contour to be achieved. The lidocaine numbs the area so no discomfort is felt, the epinephrine controls for bleeding, the cortisone controls for swelling and the bicarbonate reduces the discomfort of the injection of the solution.

- Once the area is numb the surgeon inserts a small cannula through the incision sites. The surgeon moves the cannula in a back and forth motion sucking the fat and some of the saline solution into a reservoir. In doing so numerous tunnels in the fat are created. The surrounding fat collapses into these tunnels. It is important that the surgeon leaves a small layer of fat under the skin to avoid puckering and to maintain a soft supple feel to the skin.

- When an acceptable amount of fat has been removed absorbent pads are placed over the tiny incisions and held in place by a pressure bandage which wraps around the head. This bandage is worn for 24 hours after surgery then nightly for 10 days.

- The incisions are not stitched in order to allow the excess saline solution to drain and to promote faster and better healing.

What can be expected after the surgery?

There may be some aching in the treated region after the surgery and this can be managed with an analgesic such as Tylenol. Aspirin or similar products should not be used as they promote bleeding and bruising.

Bruising with the tumescent technique is unusual, but if it occurs it will subside within 4 to 10 days. Swelling subsides within 4 days.

Most people are comfortable returning to work and being seen in public within 4 days, once the swelling subsides and the incisions sites have closed.

No change in eating behavior is required.

Will there be a scar?

The incisions are only 2 to 4 millimeters in length and are placed such that they are not obvious so that the resulting scars are not noticeable. The incisions are not sutured. They close on their own within 4 days to a fine pink line. The pinkness fades over a 4 week period.

YOUNG AS YOU LOOK

What complications may occur with tumescent liposuction of the jowls and neck?

■ *Scar:* If the incisions heal in an abnormal fashion a tiny scar may be noticeable. There are many effective ways of treating abnormal scar formation. If the scar is raised it may be flattened with an injection of cortisone. Discoloration, either red or brown, may be removed with a vascular or pigment removal laser, respectively. If the scar is depressed it may be raised with a soft tissue implant or resurfaced with the CO_2 laser.

■ *Numbness:* Alteration of sensation is very rare but if it occurs it usually is resolved within a few days.

■ *Drooping lip:* If the facial nerve is traumatized during the surgery then a permanent droop of the corner of the lip may occur. This is extremely rare and unlikely to happen.

Who performs liposuction of the jowls and neck?

Dermatologists, plastic surgeons and esthetic surgeons trained in tumescent liposuction perform this procedure on all areas of the body. The cost ranges from $2,000 to $4,000 for the jowl, cheek and neck regions. Many surgeons like to have an anaesthetist on hand to monitor vital signs so that they are able to perform the surgery without distraction. In these cases the price is higher but so is the margin of safety for the patient.

CHAPTER 9

The *Eyes*

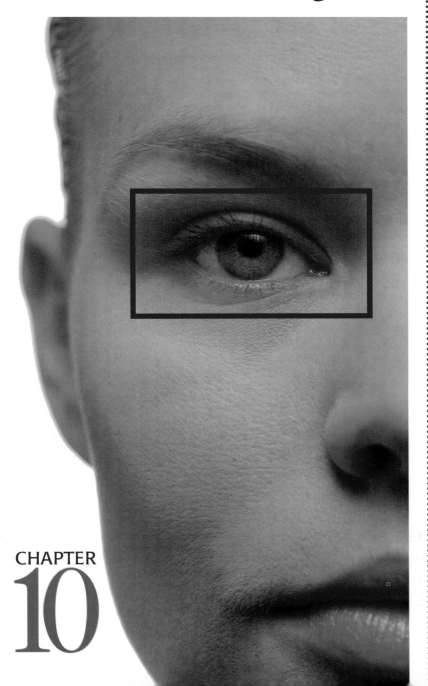

A CLEAR VIEW

The clarity of our vision frames our world. For most people the awkwardness of eye glasses or contact lenses are certainly more acceptable than poor vision.

CHAPTER
10

*Now,
however,
the evolution
of technology
and the
surgeons
skills have
made it
possible
for many to
see again
without
optical aids.*

ILLUSTRATION
COURTESY OF
GIMBEL EYE
CENTRE

Our agenda for clear
sight includes:

▌ *nearsightedness*
▌ *farsightedness*
▌ *astigmatism*
▌ *corrective surgical techniques*

Our vision is the most
significant of the senses because
75-80% of what we learn is
obtained through our eyes.

Those who do not have the
natural ability to see clearly strive
to find a way. Until the 1950's, this
meant eyeglasses and eyeglasses
meant frames. Frames can enhance
one's appearance or detract from it.
Most people, especially those
younger in age, would prefer not to
wear eyeglasses. For many people,
eyeglasses contribute to feelings of

low self-esteem and may contribute
to introverted or self-conscious
behavior.

We all remember some children
of our childhood who for reasons of
nearsightedness, farsightedness or
astigmatism had to wear eyeglasses.
Usually the unfortunate youngster
was nicknamed "four eyes". Because
of their visual difficulties they often
were required to sit near the front
of the classroom thus increasing
their conspicuousness and self-
consciousness.

In the 1950's the hard contact
lens was developed. Those who
dared to wear this revolutionary
vision enhancer suddenly regained
a freedom that they had lost when
eyeglasses became necessary, as
well as their own natural looks.
Unfortunately many people could

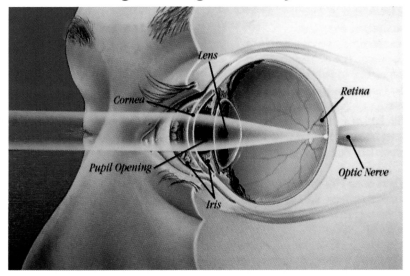

Light Entering A Normal Eye

Lens

Cornea

Retina

Pupil Opening

Optic Nerve

Iris

not tolerate these lenses and continued to require their eyeglasses.

In the early 1960's a new soft flexible plastic was developed and the soft contact lens was introduced. With it many more people were able to participate in a spectacle-free lifestyle. However, the hassle of solutions and cleaning regimes cause many people to return to the simplicity of eyeglasses.

Dr. Fyderov of Russia changed the world of the spectacle wearer. In 1975 he discovered that a person's vision could be altered by strategically placing fine incisions in the cornea, the protective lens which covers the front of the eye. This reshaped the cornea making it possible for the eye to focus without eyeglasses or contact lenses in some cases.

Since Dr. Fyderov's revolutionary discovery new surgical techniques for correcting focusing problems of the eyes have been developed. Lasers in particular have contributed to the improvement of corrective eye surgery.

With the rapid advances in laser procedures to alter the cornea of the eye, the majority of people with nearsightedness, farsightedness and astigmatism are able to achieve clear, natural vision and to be freed from the use of corrective lenses.

This means both a visual freedom as well as the cosmetic freedom to be seen as oneself without eyeglasses which alters one's appearance and self image.

Focusing Problems

The cornea is the outer lens of the eye. It is a transparent lens that covers the iris and the pupil providing protection and the eye's general focusing power. The inside lens provides the fine focusing power. For clear vision, these two lenses work together to focus light rays precisely on the retina, which is the inner back layer of the eye. The retina gathers light and picks up visual images which are then transmitted to the brain. It is like the film of a camera.

Three elements contribute to an image being in focus:

▮ the shape of the cornea,
▮ the power of the lens, and
▮ the length of the eyeball.

When all three elements are well coordinated, clear images are focused on the retina and normal vision results. However, due to hereditary and developmental factors, many eyes develop in such a way that one or more of these variables are imperfect, resulting in focussing problems.

CHAPTER

10

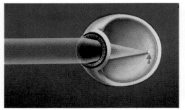
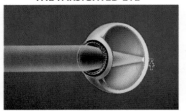
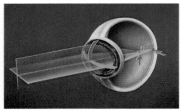

ILLUSTRATIONS
COURTESY OF
GIMBEL EYE
CENTRE

Nearsightedness

Nearsightedness, or myopia, is the most common focusing problem, affecting over 25% of the North American population. In some races this percentage is even higher.

Nearsighted people are unable to focus on distant objects but may be able to see clearly at various ranges of close objects. Therefore some form of visual correction is necessary. The condition of near-sightedness is usually hereditary and results from an eyeball that is too long. This extra length prevents light from focussing on the retina and the light rays from distant objects converge to a focal point in front of the retina. The light rays then diverge and cause a blurred image on the retina. Since the retina only captures the quality of the image that reaches it, the brain receives a blurred image of what the eye is trying to see.

Farsightedness

Farsightedness, or hyperopia, is a focusing problem caused by an eyeball that is shorter than normal. Because of the reduced length, the lenses do not have enough space in which to consistently bring light rays to a focal point by the time they reach the retina. Hence the focal point of an close object falls behind the retina resulting in a blurred image.

The effects of farsightedness vary with age because of the diminishing flexibility of the eye's inner lens. Young people may not notice the effects of mild far-sightedness because the flexibility of their inner lens allows them to adapt. But as the eyes begin to age, near objects become increasingly difficult to see. Later in life, nearly all focal ranges may be unclear.

Astigmatism

Astigmatism occurs because the cornea has more curvature in one direction or meridian than in the other. Instead of being spherical in shape like a basketball, the cornea is shaped more like a football, and this causes distortion of vision which is called astigmatism.

Nobody has a perfectly shaped cornea, but the distortion of most eyes is so slight that it does not

CHAPTER
10

significantly affect the quality of vision. However, a significant degree of astigmatism can result in major focusing problems. Astigmatism can occur by itself but often occurs in conjunction with nearsightedness and farsightedness.

Corrective Surgical Techniques

Since nearsightedness, farsightedness and astigmatism are caused by anatomical factors (too long, too short, or distortion) for most people the best way to overcome or improve their focusing abilities is to surgically alter the shape of the cornea. This is preferable to more invasive procedures because it does not involve entering the eye and because the cornea is so accessible.

For many years, since the mid 1970's, radial keratotomy (RK) and astigmatic keratotomy (AK) were the only techniques readily available to change the shape of the cornea. By use of controlled incisions on the cornea, low amounts of nearsightedness and astigmatism could be corrected. People needing moderate to high ranges of correction were left without a reliable solution until the advent of advanced laser surgery. Not only is radial keratotomy limited in its effectiveness but fluctuations in vision may occur after the surgery because the incisions penetrate 90% of the cornea, which can cause weakness of the lens.

What are the laser surgery alternatives for the correction of visual acuity?

Photorefractive Keratectomy (PRK)

Photorefractive Keratectomy (PRK) is a surgical procedure effective in correcting nearsightedness, farsightedness and astigmatism. PRK was first performed in Berlin, Germany in 1987. Since that time, hundreds of thousands of people around the world have found a new visual freedom through laser surgery.

After extensive analysis of the eye, surgeons and technicians work together to program an excimer laser to vaporize away microscopic layers of corneal tissue. With a modified curvature, focusing problems are reduced or eliminated.

The excimer laser is a unique type of "cold" laser that does not burn or cut tissue. Instead, it gently breaks the molecular bonds between cells so that controlled amounts of tissue can be literally vaporized away, one microscopic layer at a time.

When using PRK to correct nearsightedness, the curvature of the cornea is reduced centrally. For the correction of farsightedness, the tissue is reshaped on the periphery of the cornea. To correct astigmatism, more tissue is removed from some parts of the cornea than others to even out the curvature. In most cases, only 10 to 15% of the thickness of the cornea

CHAPTER

10

is removed. Eyes usually heal well, and the results are very satisfactory, with most people achieving normal or near normal natural vision.

Who Qualifies for PRK?

To be a candidate for surgery, you must meet each of the following qualifications:

- be at least 18 years of age,
- have visual acuity problems that are in a correctable range,
- have had stable vision for one year. Very slight prescription changes may be acceptable,
- have eyes free from complicating injuries and diseases, and
- must not be pregnant or nursing.

What can be expected during PRK surgery?

Each patient goes through a comprehensive series of eye tests and examinations before consulting with a surgeon to discuss and plan the specifics of personal visual correction.

During the surgery, patients sit in a reclining dentist-like chair that is lowered to a horizontal position. The degree of correction required is programmed into the laser. The eye is anaesthetized with drops, to ensure a painless experience. No injections are necessary. Once the eye is numb the eyelid is held open with a lid speculum to prevent blinking. The cornea is gently wiped then the laser light is applied. While the laser precisely vaporizes away microscopic layers of tissue, patients watch a flashing light. A soft contact lens which serves as a bandage is placed over the eye and is left in place for two days.

The actual laser surgery time is only 10 to 90 seconds depending on the amount of correction required. The total procedure takes between 10 to 15 minutes from the time the patient first enters the laser surgical suite.

Correcting Nearsightedness

ILLUSTRATIONS
COURTESY OF
GIMBEL EYE
CENTRE

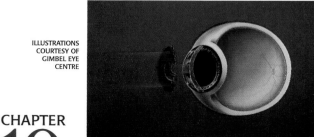

Excimer Laser Reducing Curvature
to Correct Nearsightedness

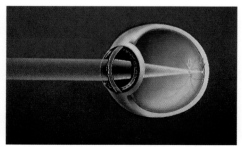

After PRK, Light Focuses
on the Retina

CHAPTER

10

Y O U N G   A S   Y O U   L O O K

What can be expected after the surgery?

As with other surgeries, recovery is a key component of the surgical process. Patients are able to walk out of the surgery suite because only local anesthesia has been used. Patients are encouraged to rest much of the next 2 days, when very significant healing occurs. Most have functional vision and can resume normal activities and work within 1 to 4 days. However, it may take several weeks for the vision to fully stabilize.

Medicated eyedrops are prescribed and are to be used for several weeks following the surgery. Patients must also diligently attend all post surgical appointments to ensure the healing and stabilization is well monitored.

Does the surgery hurt?

The surgery itself does not hurt because the eye is anaesthetized. Once the anesthetic wears off moderate discomfort of the eye is felt for 24 to 48 hours. This is managed with prescribed pain-killers such as Toradol. The contact lens bandage helps to make the eye more comfortable, as it protects it from the movement of the eyelid. It is important to keep the eye moist during the healing process as this also helps to keep the eye comfortable.

Can both eyes be treated at the same time?

It is preferable that one eye is treated at a time so that the healing process of the first eye can be observed and adjustments made for the second eye if need be. It is, however, possible for some candidates to have surgery on both eyes on the same day, conditional on the surgeon's approval and the patient's consent.

What can be done if the surgery does not turn out as expected?

If the objectives of visual correction are not met with the first surgery, a

Correcting Farsightedness

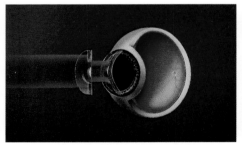

Excimer Laser Increasing Curvature to Correct Farsightedness

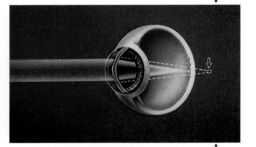

After PRK, Light Focuses on the Retina

CHAPTER
10

second, or enhancement, procedure can usually be performed to provide additional correction. Most people do not require additional surgery, but the greater the amount of correction necessary, the greater the probability that an enhancement for full correction will be necessary. The surgeon and the patient together assess the need and make the decision about further surgery.

What are the risks and side effects of PRK surgery?

As with any surgical procedure, PRK laser surgery has some possible risks and side effects that must be taken into account. Each candidate should remember that a specific end result cannot be guaranteed, although it can be closely predicted based on data from thousands of previous cases.

Serious complications are very rare. Infection is the largest risk, but its occurrence is extremely low. Even if it develops, infection can usually be cleared effectively with medications. Other possible complications include haze, ghosting, scarring, induced astigmatism, and too much or too little healing response. Most complications are treatable with medications or further surgery.

During the healing process, most people can expect to experience at least some of the following side effects:

- since small amounts of the removed tissue regenerate, the laser is programmed to take this into account and to remove enough tissue for the eye to stabilize at the desired correction, therefore, the initial effect may seem to be overcorrection,

- increased sensitivity to light,

- halo effect from bright lights at night,

- decreased visual clarity in dim light, and

- slightly drier eyes.

In most cases, these effects decrease and disappear as the eye heals. Occasionally, some may persist. Contact lenses, although rarely necessary, cannot be worn on the eye for several months following surgery.

Laser Assisted In Situ Keratomileusis (LASIK)

For some patients, a procedure called Laser In Situ Keratomileusis (LASIK) may be the best way to achieve clear, natural vision. This procedure had its origins back in the 1960's and has evolved over the years into a safe and effective operation. The current technique involves both the use of conventional and laser surgery to correct nearsightedness, farsightedness and astigmatism.

In performing LASIK surgery, the surgeon first uses a special oscillating blade to make a partial

YOUNG AS YOU LOOK

cut through 1/4 to 1/3 of the front surface of the cornea, creating a flap of clear tissue on the central part of the eye. The patient is then positioned under the excimer laser which is programmed to vaporize away some of the internal corneal tissue under the flap.

Central tissue is removed to reduce curvature and correct nearsightedness. Peripheral tissue is removed to increase curvature and correct farsightedness. Astigmatism can be corrected by removing selected tissue to even out the irregular curvature of the cornea. After the laser has removed the selected tissue, the flap is closed over the eye. The cornea has extraordinary natural bonding qualities that allow effective healing without the use of stitches. The entire procedure takes about 15 minutes, but a comprehensive examination and consultation are necessary before surgery. Patients remain awake with only the designated eye anaesthetized with drops. Good vision is often possible on the day following the surgery. Eye drops and night protection are necessary for a period of time.

Does the surgery hurt?

LASIK surgery is more comfortable post-operatively than PRK surgery because the corneal flap covers and protects the area treated. However, because of the intricacy of the

surgery it tends to be reserved for people who require a significant amount of correction.

What are the risks and side effects of LASIK surgery?

Possible risks of LASIK surgery include:

- Creating a cap of corneal tissue instead of just a flap by fully removing the top of the cornea rather than just lifting it. This removed tissue still heals back into place but requires extra care in positioning.

- Infection is very rare and is controlled with medications.

- Epithelial tissue growth underneath the flap can usually be solved by lifting the flap and gently removing these tissue cells.

- Increased or decreased response to surgery can usually be modified by lifting the cap and removing more tissue with the laser. Sometimes other types of surgery can be combined with LASIK to give improved results.

Side effects are minimal following LASIK surgery since most of the surface of the cornea has not been affected by the procedure. But people who have the surgery may experience some light sensitivity and glare for a few days or weeks. Full visual stabilization may take several weeks.

CHAPTER
10

What are the benefits of laser eye surgery?

Most patients achieve the desired correction for their visual acuity problems and are happy to be free to work, to play, to live without eyeglasses or contact lenses.

It means their own true facial features and eyes are not altered or cosmetically compromised by the need for corrective lenses.

With the speed and accuracy of laser surgery patients can gain freedom from eyeglasses, enhance their appearance, enjoy the possibilities of career choices that require good natural vision, and be freed from all the clutter that is associated with contact lenses.

Who performs surgical techniques to correct visual acuity problems and how much does it cost?

Opthalmologists with special training in these techniques perform the surgery for $2,000 to $3,000 per eye.

CHAPTER
10

The *Teeth*

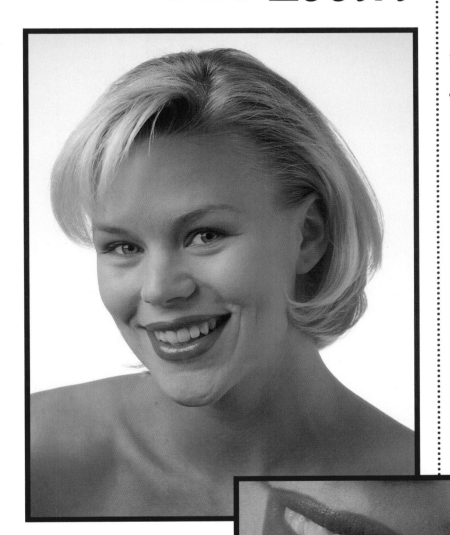

THE POWER OF THE SMILE

*Teeth were
meant to last
a lifetime,
and with
daily care,
and regular
visits to
the dentist,
they should.*

11 CHAPTER

Unfortunately,

tooth loss can

still occur,

but thanks

to modern

technology

and dental

techniques,

the quality

and comfort

level of

replacement

teeth has risen

dramatically

in the

last decade.

As with

other parts of

our body,

the growth of

our teeth

does not

always follow

defined paths.

Yellowed or discolored teeth detract from a pleasant smile. Cosmetic dentistry provides you with many solutions to these perplexing problems.

Our agenda for a more attractive smile includes:

- *gum disease*
- *discolored teeth*
- *veneers*
- *crowns*
- *fractured or chipped teeth*
- *worn teeth*
- *lost teeth*
- *crooked teeth*

Personalities in the media with what appear to be perfectly straight, white teeth are constant reminders of the power of a smile. A smile is able to suggest warmth and beauty and reveal one's state of health. If teeth and gums are healthy, the smile can be beautiful.

Increasingly, dentists are being asked about problems associated with cosmetics and aging. The list of potential problems associated with teeth is long and includes teeth that are:

- discolored
- worn
- chipped
- missing
- misaligned.

The victim of these problems wants to smile again without embarrassment or discomfort.

The shape and color of teeth may be altered through bonding or with crowns. Missing teeth can be replaced by fixed or removable bridges, or dentures. Tooth alignment can be altered using orthodontics (braces). Facial features are sometimes dramatically altered with orthognathic surgery.

There are ways to keep your smile healthy and beautiful and to alter and reverse those changes caused by either neglect or aging. Options for enhancing the smile are impressive. This area should not be ignored as you strive to look as young as you feel.

GUMS

No matter how nice the teeth look, if the gums are unhealthy deterioration will set in and lead to tooth loss. Gum (periodontal) disease is the number one reason for tooth loss in the adult population.

Periodontal disease is caused by bacteria (plaque) growing on the teeth. A substance the bacteria releases causes the gums to become infected. If the bacteria are not removed, the bone under the gums becomes infected, resulting in bone loss. Eventually the tooth has so little bone holding it in place that it becomes loose and may have to be pulled.

Since the process is slow and insidious, it is important to recognize the early signs of periodontal disease and to have the gums checked regularly.

The gums are normally a coral pink color. One of the first signs of gum disease is red gums that bleed. If the gums bleed during normal, regular brushing or flossing, the problem is gum disease and requires a dentist's assistance to remedy.

How can gum disease be prevented?

The good news is that gum disease may be prevented by proper daily tooth care. It is more important to brush and floss the teeth thoroughly once a day (preferably before bedtime) than quickly and poorly three times a day. Proper cleaning should take from 5 to 10 minutes. If any problems are experienced with brushing and flossing, they should be discussed with a dentist.

Brushing

The best technique for brushing is as follows:

- Use a soft brush with single tufts in 2 or 3 rows.

- Brush systematically: start on one side of the mouth, going completely around the teeth to the other side. Then, brush the inside of the teeth from one side to the next.

- The brush should be angled at 45 degrees to the tooth with the bristles contacting the bottom

third of the tooth. The brush is moved in short rotary strokes, cleaning 1 or 2 teeth at a time.

- Brushing will remove plaque only from the outside and inside surfaces of the teeth. In order to remove the plaque from between the teeth, they must be flossed.

Dental floss

There are two types of floss: waxed and unwaxed. Unwaxed floss cleans teeth better, but if the floss shreds between the teeth, use waxed floss.

- A 30 to 45 centimeter (12 to 18 inch) length of floss is wrapped around the middle finger of one hand and positioned over the tips of the index fingers.

- The index fingers should be about 2 1/2 centimeters (1 inch) apart and the floss is worked between the teeth with a slight back and forth shoe shining motion, until it passes through the contact points between the teeth.

- The floss is then wrapped around the tooth, forming a C-shape, and moved up and down the tooth surface. Once one surface is cleaned, it can be wrapped around the other tooth surface to be cleaned. The floss should then be pulled out from between the teeth. The same procedure is repeated for all teeth.

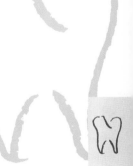

11 CHAPTER

TEETH

There are two types of stains that can discolor the teeth. One is called extrinsic: stains caused by substances sticking directly to the surface of the teeth. The most common causes are coffee, tea, and smoking. Extrinsic stains cannot be removed by regular brushing. A regular professional cleaning done by a hygienist or dentist will remove the stains along with any associated bacteria.

The other type of stain is intrinsic or within the tooth. The most common intrinsic staining is characterized by white or yellow spots and sometimes by bands on the teeth. These are usually caused by old fillings that start to leak or change color. Intrinsic discoloration may also form while the tooth is developing. Certain medications may contribute to this problem. The antibiotic tetracycline taken during the years that the teeth are developing will cause the teeth to have a yellowish-grey color. It is for this reason that pregnant mothers and children under 9 years of age should not take tetracycline, if at all possible. Some illnesses, when accompanied by a high fever, will also cause this discoloration.

If a tooth starts to turn darker than the adjacent teeth, the cause is likely an abscess or a tooth that has had a root canal treatment. The discoloration is caused by blood inside the tooth being incorporated into the tooth structure. With time, these pigments will move closer to the surface of the tooth, turning it even darker.

To change the inherent color of your teeth or to correct an internal stain a bleaching gel can be applied daily. The length of time that the gel is left on the tooth and the frequency of use determines the response that is obtained. It is expected that there will be some improvement within a month of daily application. The bleach will not change the color of existing fillings or crowns. So if these blend with the color of the teeth before bleaching they will not blend afterwards.

The bleaching gel is placed in a splint to keep the gel in proximity to the teeth. It is possible to target one or two teeth that are particularly discolored by strategically placing the gel in the splint. Sensitivity of the gums or teeth to the gel may result in the gel having to be discontinued or limited in use.

A more recent technique for tackling internal discoloration of the teeth is the use of a bleaching gel in combination with a CO_2 or Nd:YAG laser. The gel is applied to the teeth and a laser light is used to encourage absorbtion into the enamel of the tooth. As this technique is relatively new it is not known what the long term effects on the tooth will be. There may be some risk that the tooth could be damaged in the process.

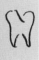

11 CHAPTER

182   *Y O U N G   A S   Y O U   L O O K*

015012

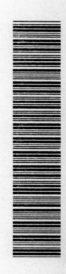

MARTINEZ JAVIER
97 POPLAR STREET
JERSEY CITY
07307-3231

NJ

STATE OF NEW JERSEY

2002 INCOME TAX REFUND

MARTINEZ JAVIER
97 POPLAR STREET
JERSEY CITY   NJ
07307-3231

CHECK NUMBER: J   210976614
CHECK DATE: MARCH 06,2003
CHECK AMOUNT: 136.00

DLN: 308875929

TAX04P (Rev 1/18/2002)

DETACH BEFORE CASHING CHECK AND RETAIN AS EVIDENCE OF PAYMENT

The dentist also is able to apply a composite bond, a veneer, or a crown to cover intrinsic discoloration. Each of these processes has advantages and disadvantages.

Composite Bonds

Composite bonding is another method of restoring the color of the teeth. The composite used is filling material composed of a resin or plastic-like material. Bonding is the manner in which this material is adhered to the tooth.

A composite comes in various shades which a skilled dentist is trained to match to the teeth thus providing the proper color and contour. For substantially dis-colored teeth, composite bonding may not be effective in masking the stain and still maintain a natural look, but for minor discolorations, it works well.

The following are the steps the dentist takes in composite bonding:

- The correct color is selected to match the surrounding teeth.

- The tooth is cleaned and the surface prepared with drilling. Since this preparation involves the surface of the tooth, local anesthetic is not necessary in most cases.

- The tooth is then "etched" with a mild acid to provide a surface to which the composite will bond.

- Mouldable composite filling

material is used and a high-intensity light is placed on the tooth for about 40 seconds to harden the composite.

- The composite is refined and polished.

What are the advantages and disadvantages of bonding?

The advantages of composite bonding are low cost, little or no anesthesia is required, it is relatively easy to reverse, there is minimal loss of natural tooth structure, a dramatic result can be achieved in a short period of time, and it is reasonably durable.

The disadvantages, however, are that the composite bonded tooth may discolor over time, break, and may have to be replaced in five years. Composite bonding is not effective in completely covering darkly colored imperfections.

What does it cost?

Depending on the dentist and his or her location, the cost will vary between $75 and $200 per tooth.

Veneers

As the name implies, veneering is the placement of a thin facing over the front surface of a tooth. These facings are made of either resin or porcelain. The technique is similar to the placement of a composite bond. Facings, unlike composites, are fabricated in the laboratory.

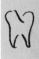

Two visits to the dentist are required for this procedure. During the first appointment, between 0.25 and 0.50 millimeter of tooth structure is removed from the front surface of the tooth, and an imprint is made of it. The facings are fitted and adjusted during the next visit. At this time, the tooth surface is etched with a mild acid to create a surface to which the facing will bond. A resin is then used to adhere the facing to the tooth.

What are the advantages and disadvantages of veneers?

The advantages are that a minimal amount of tooth structure is removed, it is esthetically pleasing, and the veneer is replaceable should it become damaged, providing that enough tooth structure remains underneath.

The disadvantages are that the tooth is thicker due to the addition of the facing, the veneer may chip, fracture, or come loose, and it lasts only about five years.

How much does a veneer cost?

The cost ranges from $200 to $500 per tooth.

Crowns

Crowning or capping is the process by which the entire surface of the tooth is removed and replaced with a covering (or crown) made of porcelain and occasionally bonded to gold.

Two appointments are needed. During the first visit, the dentist removes about one millimeter of tooth structure. An imprint of the tooth is then taken, so that a model from which the crown is fabricated can be made. Next, the prepared tooth is covered with a temporary restoration to last until the second visit. The permanent crown is fitted to the tooth on the second visit. Adjustments are made for shape and color so the crown matches the natural teeth. It is then permanently cemented onto the tooth.

What are the advantages and disadvantages of crowns?

The advantages are that the shade can be altered as desired; overall tooth shape can be changed; and the result is esthetically pleasing.

The disadvantages are as follows: crowning involves the removal of a considerable amount of tooth structure and is, therefore, not reversible; as the color of the adjacent teeth changes with time, the crown does not change, resulting in a mismatch between the natural teeth and the bond; if the gums shrink, an unsightly line might be visible at the gum line; the life expectancy of a crown is 5 to 20 years; and longer dental appointments are needed than for bonding.

How expensive are crowns?

Crowning or capping is the most expensive procedure for improving tooth color. It will cost between $400 and $1,500 per crown.

Fractured or Chipped Teeth

Teeth are relatively fragile and, if traumatized, often will chip or fracture. If the fracture does not involve the pulp (the inside of the tooth), the solution may be to bond the tooth. If the pulp is damaged, however, it will be necessary to undergo a root canal operation or the tooth will likely abscess. Due to this possible complication, it is important that no permanent treatment, such as a crown, be applied to a recently traumatized tooth.

To restore a chipped tooth, the dentist first determines if any pulp has been damaged. If so, then a root canal is necessary. This involves cleaning out the canal inside the root which carries the nerves and blood vessels.

If no pulpal damage exists, the dentist will determine if there is enough tooth structure left to bond the tooth. If there is, composite bonding may be applied. If there is not enough tooth structure for bonding, it may be necessary to place pins into the tooth to hold the composite bonding in place. After a 3 month period, the tooth is re-evaluated to determine if the pulp is still healthy and whether more definitive treatment, such as a crown, is necessary.

Worn Teeth

With age, the teeth wear and the biting edges of the front teeth are flattened, making them shorter and all of the same length. Eventually, less and less tooth is displayed, giving an aged look to the mouth.

Generally, the teeth wear slowly, but if a person grinds the teeth (bruxism) wear can be rapid and the amount of tooth worn away may be extensive. Although bruxism is a common problem, it rarely causes tooth loss.

If teeth are worn down, the cause needs to be established. If it is due to a tooth being out of position, it should be corrected. If it is due to bruxism, a removable acrylic splint which covers the teeth should be worn.

Solutions to improving worn teeth are the application of crowns or, if wear is minimal, composite bonding.

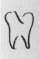

Gaps

Few procedures in dentistry make a more dramatic difference than the closure of spaces between teeth. Spaces frequently result from a discrepancy between the size of the teeth and the size of the jaw. They may also be due to the loss of a tooth or teeth, which allows the other teeth to shift and thus open up spaces.

The most common area for a gap is between the two front teeth. If this gap is no larger than

2 millimeters (1/32 of an inch), the space can be closed with composite bonding. If it is larger, orthodontics, veneers, crowns, or a combination of these approaches needs to be considered.

If the gap is due to tooth loss, the tooth needs to be replaced with a fixed bridge. The space is bridged by crowning the teeth on either side of the space and connecting them with a false tooth. The bridge is cemented over the adjacent teeth and does not come out.

Another alternative is a removable bridge which does not require crowning of adjacent teeth. The removable bridge is held in place by wire clasps around the teeth on either side of the space, but is not as comfortable or as easy to care for as is the fixed bridge. If there are too many missing teeth, however, and the remaining teeth are loose, a removable bridge may have to be used.

To maintain the overall health of the mouth, a lost tooth must be replaced. Teeth are maintained in position by each other. Therefore, if one tooth is lost, the teeth behind the space will tilt forward and the teeth in the opposite jaw will move into the space. With time, these changes affect the bite and cause the loss of other teeth as well. If numerous back teeth are missing, the bite may close down. This could contribute to the formation of wrinkles around the mouth, and thus premature aging in a younger adult.

Fixed bridges have certain advantages. They improve the bite, maintain the position of the teeth, and improve the appearance. The disadvantage of a fixed bridge is that some tooth structure must be forfeited in order for the supporting crowns to be placed on the adjacent teeth. A fixed bridge lasts anywhere from 5 to 20 years and costs between $400 and $1,200 per tooth.

Missing Teeth

Dentures

When all the teeth have been lost, they are replaced with a complete set of dentures. It is a mistake, however, to believe that once dentures are in place, there are no longer any problems and therefore no need to see the dentist regularly. Complete dentures present problems, such as decreased chewing ability, decreased sense of taste, sore spots, and difficulty in keeping the dentures in place. They may cause embarrassment if they fall out at an awkward moment.

The bone the dentures rest on continually and irreversibly resorbs or deteriorates, affecting the placement of the dentures on the ridges. Therefore, it is important to visit the dentist regularly to build up areas of wear on the dentures.

YOUNG AS YOU LOOK

What complications might dentures cause?

Several complications are associated with dentures, including a collapsed profile, too much or too little tooth display, inadequate lip support, and a resorption of the bone which supports the denture.

If the chin and nose seem to come closer together when biting, a collapsed profile may be the problem. As denture teeth and ridges of the jaw wear, the lower jaw has to close further for the teeth to meet. This results in a collapsed and aged looking profile. Persistent sores in the corner of the mouth may also be a problem. The solution is to make new dentures with the teeth set so that the jaw closes at the level it once did, restoring the profile to its proper vertical dimension.

Worn denture teeth may result in very little display of the teeth when smiling. The solution is to replace the denture teeth with new ones. In contrast, if dentures are too big they look like they are falling out and the gums show while smiling. Denture teeth need to be reset in a correct position, which often entails the making of a new denture.

If the lips feel as if they are caving in, and seem to have more wrinkles, the cause may be inadequate lip support by the denture. The denture needs to be remade with a thicker flange (gum portion), and the teeth need to be placed further forward.

Another complication with dentures is that they may move around in the mouth or even fall out. This happens because the remaining bone continually resorbs once the natural teeth are removed. Over time, less and less bone remains to hold the dentures in place. As a consequence, the dentures start to move around. The first step is to have the dentures relined or remade. If this does not provide satisfactory retention or function, implants are considered as the next step.

Implants

Implants are a means of securing a denture or bridge to the bone. Implants are placed into the jaw bone and the bridge is fixed onto the implant. There are many different implant systems, but the osseointegrated (joined bone) system has the highest success rate, is the most predictable, and rarely fails.

How are dental implants placed?

The steps involved in an implant are as follows:

- In the jaw bone, 4 to 6 small titanium fixtures resembling screws are implanted. The procedure takes about 2 hours and is performed under local or general anesthetic.

- Over a period of 3 to 6 months, the jaw bone fuses to these titanium fixtures, forming a stable biological bond. This process is called osseointegration.

Dental Implants

BEFORE

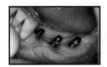

AFTER

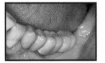

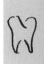

11 CHAPTER

- After this biological bonding has occurred, titanium abutments are attached to the fixtures. This second stage of the surgical procedure takes about 1 hour.

- About 2 weeks later, impressions, bite registrations, tooth selections, and bridge fittings are undertaken.

- Finally, a fixed bridge is attached to the abutments with gold screws. The final bridge requires the same care given to natural teeth.

What are the advantages and disadvantages of dental implants?

The ability to chew foods properly and efficiently without discomfort is the most important advantage. As well, there is no longer concern over losing a denture at an awkward moment. The cost, however, is high. The surgical portion alone will cost between $5,000 to $7,000 and the bridge another $5,000 to $7,000. In addition, the success rate is not 100%. Implants occasionally fail and have to be removed. In some cases, titanium fixtures may be visible at the gum line when smiling.

Crooked Teeth

Ever increasing numbers of adults are undergoing orthodontic treatment for poorly aligned teeth, crowding, cross bites, and missing or crooked teeth. Cosmetic surgery is not a substitute for orthodontics but should be harmonized with orthodontics and other dental care to achieve an esthetically pleasing result.

The orthodontist adjusts tooth alignment using braces to obtain an acceptable bite and an esthetically pleasing smile. The steps involved are as follows:

- A complete diagnosis of the problem is the first step.

- Preliminary dental work, including restorative work, fillings, and gum tissue therapy must be completed before braces can be applied. Some tooth extraction may be necessary before braces are fitted on the teeth.

- Braces are placed, and a series of scheduled adjustments are made during the time the braces are worn. The newer braces are less obvious than the "mouth of metal" worn in the past. The length of time the braces are worn varies according to the extent of the realignment required.

- The braces are removed and a retainer is provided to control tooth movement. It may be necessary to wear this over a period of 3 to 18 months.

Depending on the extent of procedure necessary, braces cost anywhere from $2,500 to $5,500.

YOUNG AS YOU LOOK

THE JAWS

Painful Jaw Joint

The relationship between dental occlusion (the bite) and temporomandibular (jaw) joint symptoms is highly controversial. Orthodontics are sometimes helpful in relieving discomfort but cannot be relied upon to correct this problem. Braces, mouth splints, and other techniques may be helpful. Symptoms such as pain, headaches, and clicking may seem to go away while braces are on, but they often return once the braces are removed.

The cost of these techniques can vary depending on the extent of the procedure necessary.

Poorly Positioned Jaws

Severe malocclusion, a condition in which the jaws and therefore the teeth do not line up properly, is uncommon, especially in adults. This problem cannot be camouflaged or modified by growth changes and ultimately requires several therapeutic steps, including restorative dentistry, realignment of the teeth, and surgical repositioning of the jaw or teeth. To accomplish this, a comprehensive diagnosis of the problem and a treatment schedule is necessary so that all the professionals involved are working toward the same goal.

There are four basic ways to correct the jaw (also called orthognathic surgery), and they are performed as follows:

Lower jaw advancement:
This is one of the most common oral surgery procedures performed today. The goal is to lengthen the lower jaw so that it aligns properly with the nose, resulting in a more attractive profile. Several surgical techniques may be used to accomplish this goal and the oral surgeon will determine the best technique to suit each individual's needs. Generally, these surgical interventions are intra-oral (done inside the mouth). No scar will be visible.

Lower jaw set back:
An excessively large lower jaw is rare in the overall population (3% in Caucasians). It may be accompanied by problems with the upper jaw. The surgical procedures for moving the lower jaw back into alignment with the upper vary according to the needs of the individual. Again, the incisions are intra-oral.

Upper jaw adjustments:
It is possible to move the upper jaw (or maxilla) upward, downward, backward, and forward, as well as to increase or decrease the width, all to varying degrees. Adjustments are frequently made in conjunction with lower jaw surgery, although sometimes it may only be necessary to modify the chin's appearance by inserting a silastic implant as discussed in the chapter Facial

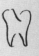

11 CHAPTER

Harmony. The incisions are intra-oral.

Combined upper and lower jaw surgery:

Depending on the individual skeletal relationships, combined surgery of the upper and lower jaw with possible chin modification may be necessary.

How is orthognathic surgery accomplished?

The sequence of events in orthognathic surgery is as follows:

■ The oral surgeon, orthodontist, and if necessary, a restorative specialist will first make a complete diagnosis of the problem. The concerns and needs of the patient will be discussed and taken into consideration, since orthognathic surgery can be a long, involved, and expensive commitment.

■ A treatment plan and schedule are developed to coordinate all the professionals involved. The plan, along with all the potential benefits and risks, is thoroughly discussed with the patient.

■ After the patient has made the decision to proceed with the designated course of treatment, all preliminary and necessary dental work is performed, including restorative work,

gum tissue therapy, and temporomandibular joint therapy.

■ The orthodontic work is then begun, and the patient is fitted with braces.

■ Oral surgery is performed next, usually requiring a hospital stay of 3 to 5 days. Once the patient leaves the hospital, he or she is provided with appropriate medication and oral hygiene and dietary instructions. It is usually necessary to take 2 to 5 weeks off work, depending on the extent of the surgery and the fixation technique used. Fixation is used to immobilize the jaw segments until healing has taken place.

■ Once the jaw has satisfactorily healed, the fixation device is removed, retainers are put in place, and physiotherapy, to strengthen and lengthen the jaw muscle and joint function, is initiated.

■ Orthodontic treatment is then completed and the braces removed. Retainers to stabilize movement of the teeth are put in place and will have to be worn for 3 to 18 months after completion of the procedure.

Y O U N G   A S   Y O U   L O O K

When is orthognathic surgery usually done?

As noted earlier, orthognathic surgery is meant for those who respond poorly to orthodontics alone and whose problem is too severe to camouflage. As a general rule, surgery is delayed until skeletal growth is complete, although surgery may be required at an earlier age if a definite growth deficiency exists. It will not, however, be performed before adolescence.

What problems might arise after orthognathic surgery?

The complications associated with orthognathic surgery include: poor union between the bones, post-operative infection, damage to the nerves resulting in numbness of the lips or tongue, temporomandibular joint problems, gum-tissue problems, unacceptable changes in facial appearance (such as a flaring of the nostrils, a potential complication with upper jaw surgery), and damage to blood vessels resulting in soft tissue and bone loss.

Who performs orthognathic surgery and what does it cost?

Oral surgeons perform surgery on the jaw and orthodontists realign the teeth. Other professionals, such as dentists, periodontists, and physiotherapists, may also be involved in the procedure.

Depending on the extent of surgery and coordinated post surgical dental care required, it can cost between $5,000 and $8,000.

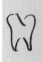

11CHAPTER

The *Hair*

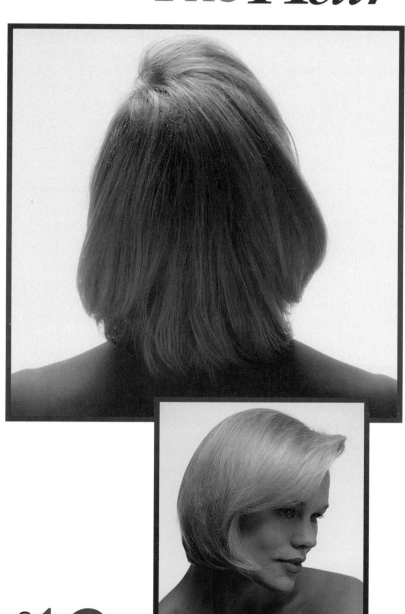

When considering appearance, two of the biggest concerns people have are superfluous hair and hair loss.

CHAPTER **12**

Today, there are numerous methods, both chemical and surgical, to correct both problems.

Our agenda for hair includes:

- *superfluous hair*
- *hair loss*
- *surgical procedures for restoring hair*
- *camouflaging hair loss*

Hair changes with age like the skin. Three changes in hair growth occur with time: going grey, growing more hair than is wanted, and/or losing hair. Greying hair, as has already been discussed, may simply be "washed away" with various rinses or dye solutions. Too much or too little hair is not dealt with quite as easily.

SUPERFLUOUS HAIR

The intensity of the battle against unwanted hair is cultural to a certain extent. For example many women in mediterranean regions are unconcerned with body hair, whereas their middle eastern neighbours laboriously pluck all the hair from their body. In North America it is estimated that consumers spend $1 billion dollars a year on electrolysis alone.

The first step in solving the dilemma of excess or unwanted hair is to determine its cause. If the problem is not medical then once

again lasers are leading the way to new and more effective ways of eliminate unwanted hair. Other more traditional methods of hair removal include electrolysis, waxing, shaving, plucking or chemical depilatories. A combination of the techniques may be the most ideal approach depending on the goals of the individual. The alternative to removing unwanted hair is camouflage by bleaching.

Laser Hair Removal

How do lasers remove hair?

There are currently two techniques being used to remove unwanted hair with laser. The first technique utilizes a new generation of Alexandrite, and ruby lasers which have a long pulse duration. These lasers have an affinity for pigment in the hair root and on application the productivity of the hair root is decreased. The hair root is stunned into a prolonged sleeping phase of up to eight months or more. When the hair root wakes up it has been weakened and may not be capable of further growth. A single treatment with the Alexandrite or Ruby lasers may be enough to eradicate fine, dark hairs. If hairs are light in color, thick or deep they may require multiple sessions or they may not respond at all.

Other photo optic light sources which are similar to lasers are also being used in a similar fashion to remove hair. Although they are not lasers they are often referred to as such.

The second technique utilizes one of four lasers: the Q-switched short pulse duration ruby, the Alexandrite, the Nd:Yag or the variable pulse width (VPW) green lasers. These lasers have an affinity for darker pigment. To attract the laser light to the hair follicles a black carbon gel is spread over the skin then wiped off. Some of this gel remains in the pores of the hair follicles. When the laser light is applied it passes harmlessly through the skin and is selectively absorbed by the dark pigment of the carbon gel. The energy emitted by the laser light when it is absorbed causes the carbon molecules to break into minuscule particles. The heat transmitted in this process damages or destroys the adjacent hair follicles. The hair growth in the treated area is significantly reduced or in many cases is completely eradicated. More than one session is usually required to achieve the desired results. The Thermolase hair removal system utilizes this technique and has been approved for this purpose by the Food and Drug Administration in the United States.

Response to either method of laser removal is variable depending on the type of hair, the color of the hair and the depth of the hair root. No assurances can be made as everyone responds differently. For this reason a test site is recommended before proceeding with extensive therapy.

Potential complications exist with all forms of hair removal. Failure to respond to the laser light, pigment changes in the skin, or even scar, could occur, although the risk is low. Allergic reactions to the gel may occur if the second technique is used. One would expect inflammation in the hair follicles for approximately ten days after the procedure.

Electrolysis

Electrolysis is a hair removal technique where, an electrical current is passed into the hair follicle, rendering it inactive and causing the hair to fall out. Currently, three methods of electrolysis are used: galvanic current, electrocoagulation, and radio wave. Each differs in the amount of time the procedure takes and the number of hairs that can be removed. The galvanic method is the slowest. Claims have been made that radio wave electrolysis is less uncomfortable and causes fewer pigmentary problems; this, however, has not yet been adequately substantiated.

The galvanic current appliances have been adapted for home use (for example, Permatweez), and although it is a slow, tedious process, for many this is preferable to going for regular, and sometimes costly, sessions at a salon.

An electrolysis program is a long-term commitment and it is often uncomfortable. Topical

CHAPTER 12

anesthetic creams can help minimize the discomfort. Possible complications include scarring, irregular pigmentation, infection, and flare-ups of acne and herpes simplex (cold sores) in the area being treated.

For these reasons it is important to be treated by a properly trained and experienced electrologist. Some geographic locations have licensing bodies for electrologists; most, however, do not. It is best therefore, to speak to a knowledgeable physician or to request references before starting a course of treatment with an unknown technician.

Other Hair Removal Techniques

Waxing

Waxing is really a way of plucking a lot of hairs at one time. Warm wax is applied to the area of hair to be removed. It cools and is pulled away from the skin, taking the trapped hair with it. Irritation often accompanies this procedure and is due to either the actual plucking or to the warm wax. This subsides within a few hours to a couple of days leaving a smooth, hairless surface for several weeks. Regrowth occurs within 5 to 9 weeks. Prior to rewaxing, the hair must grow in to above the skin surface for the wax to adhere to it. This temporary period of new hair growth might be socially uncomfortable.

During the regrowth period ingrown hairs may be troublesome. If so, run hot water over an old toothbrush to soften the bristles, then brush the skin twice daily in those areas. This helps lift the curved, irritating hair tips out of the skin and, minimizes the problem.

Repeat waxing over a period of time weakens the hair follicle and gradually reduces the amount of hair growth in the area waxed.

Rotating Coil Appliances

As with waxing, this is another form of diffuse plucking. Small rotating coils catch the hairs and pull them out by the root. The advantages of this device are that there is complete control over how much or how little is plucked and the effect lasts longer than techniques like shaving. An example of this appliance is Epilady.

Shaving

A common misconception about shaving is that the more hair is shaved, the thicker it becomes. A typical hair shaft is wider in the middle than at the ends and when it is cut off, it will appear thicker and coarser. The hair becomes coarser as the body ages. Therefore, after shaving for a long time, the hair is thicker, not because of shaving, but because of the aging process. Although women find shaving an acceptable method for getting rid of unwanted hair on some parts of the body such as the

CHAPTER 12

legs, it is not acceptable for other body parts, particularly the face.

Are there any other mechanical removal techniques?

Tweezing, plucking, pumice stones, and sandpaper-like gloves are some of the other techniques available. Pumice stones and sandpaper-like gloves are used to remove fine, excessive facial hair but can be irritating to the skin.

Tweezing and plucking are commonly used to trim and shape the eyebrows and to remove isolated hairs, for example hair in moles and around the nipples, but it can cause inflamed and infected pustules. A small dab of Fucidin antibiotic ointment applied after plucking can prevent infection. If this is a persistent problem, it may be preferable to cut the undesirable hair off flush with the skin, using scissors or a razor.

Occasionally, repetitive tweezing may result in enough damage to the hair follicle that the hair will die and no longer present a problem.

Chemical Depilatories

Some examples of chemical depilatories include Neet, Nudit, and Nair. These products break down the strong sulphur bonds that hold proteins in the hair together. The hair becomes soft and weak and can usually be wiped away. Unfortunately, the skin in the area of the unwanted hair often becomes irritated with this technique. Subsequent inflammation may stimulate the pigment cells to produce more melanin resulting in darker skin in the area (post-inflammatory pigmentation). To prevent these problems the instructions for the use of the depilatory should be followed carefully, and it should first be tested on a small area.

A dermatologist could prescribe a mild cortisone cream to apply immediately after using depilatories to prevent skin irritation and hyperpigmentation (darkening). If darkening does occur, bleaching creams such as Reversa HQ and NeoStrata HQ may be used to lighten the skin again.

Camouflage

Bleaching or dyeing unwanted hair is the best camouflaging technique but like chemical depilatories, this process may be irritating to the skin.

What if excess hair is due to hormonal imbalance?

Unwanted hair in certain parts of the body, may be due to an excess of androgens or to an over sensitivity to the normal level of androgens in the body.

If the underlying cause is a hormonal imbalance due to a tumor, the tumor must be surgically removed. If, however, the hormonal imbalance is due to other reasons, such as certain types of drugs, an overproduction of androgens (male hormones), or hyper sensitivity to normal amounts of androgens, the following prescription medications may be used to control unwanted hair:

■ *Marvelon and Demulen:* These oral contraceptive are best used for the combined problem of acne and excess hair. Its advantage in these circumstances is that it does not contain any substances related to androgen nor can it be broken down into androgen products by the body. Positive results are usually seen after 9 to 12 months of continual use.

■ *Aldactone (spironolactone):* This medication is a water pill, or diuretic, which is frequently prescribed to reduce body fluid. It has also, however, been effective in controlling unwanted hair, even when hormonal levels are relatively normal. The usual method of use is to start taking small daily doses and gradually increase them. Patients taking Aldactone are also instructed to drink 16 ounces of water or other fluids a day. It takes 9 to 12 months to see positive results. Dryness of the eyes and mouth, and an increased need to urinate, may be experienced. As the dose is increased, some women may experience irregularity in the menstrual cycle. When prescribed for men, this medication may cause thickening of the breasts. Another disadvantage is that it may have the opposite effect and actually increase hair growth.

In fact, Aldactone is sometimes prescribed for women who have male pattern hair loss to prevent such loss and to encourage hair growth.

■ *Androcur (cyproterone):* This medication is known as a progestational agent and has some anti-androgen properties. Because of these properties, it should be taken with oral birth control pills, preferably Marvelon or Demulen, or it could affect a developing fetus. It should not be used for 2 months prior to attempting pregnancy nor should it be taken by those with liver or kidney problems. It is started at a small dose and is gradually increased to a larger dose as the tolerance level improves. Positive results are usually seen in 6 to 12 months.

■ *Euflex (flutamide):* This oral medication is effective in the treatment of excess hair. By blocking the action of the male hormone, it decreases hair growth on the face and body, yet thickens the hair on the scalp. It takes about 7 to 24 months before these changes occur. It can not be given to men because of its influence on the male hormones. Flushing, dry skin, decreased libido, breast discomfort, and nausea are some of the potential side effects of this medication. There is also the risk of liver disease so careful monitoring is essential.

CHAPTER 12

198 *YOUNG AS YOU LOOK*

HAIR LOSS

Contrary to general belief the unremitting loss of hair as time passes is not restricted to the male gender. Women may also be predisposed to male pattern hair loss, although it is not as common.

Male pattern hair loss occurs when, due to a hereditary predisposition, the hair follicles are overly sensitive to normal male hormone levels and effectively burn out. Less commonly male hormones may be in excess.

Thyroid abnormalities or hormonal imbalance may unmask male pattern hair loss in both sexes, but more commonly in women. Therefore it is important to check for these conditions before embarking on a course of treatment.

Age related hair loss may be alleviated by medication, surgery, or camouflage.

Treating Hair Loss with Minoxidil

A medication, known as minoxidil, has provided the first really promising topical solution for the treatment of hair loss. Minoxidil is a drug given in tablet form to treat high blood pressure and has the side effect of hair growth on various parts of the body. Researchers applied the drug to the skin to determine whether it would have the same effect on hair growth when used externally as it does when taken internally. The results were positive.

Although minoxidil increases blood circulation to the hair follicles experts are not convinced that this is how the drug really works. There has been some suggestion that minoxidil may work by prolonging the growth phase of the hair root and preventing its shrinkage over time.

Rogaine, Apogaine, and Minoxigaine are the only products currently available that contain minoxidil to encourage hair growth on the scalp. Prior to the availability of Rogaine and its successors, some forward thinking dermatologists were having pharmacists grind minoxidil pills into a base for application to the scalp. The advantage of pharmaceutical mixtures over this method is that it is a standardized formula which has the same amount of all the ingredients in each prescription.

Recent studies suggest that using tretinoin (Retin-A, Stieva-A, Vitamin A Acid, Renova, Retisol-A, Rejuva-A) in combination with minoxidil may speed up the process of regrowth by encouraging better penetration by the minoxidil, but more research is necessary to substantiate these findings.

Does minoxidil work for everyone who is balding?

In studies where hundreds of men used minoxidil, not everyone with male pattern baldness responded by

CHAPTER 12

growing hair. Some grew noticeable amounts of hair, others grew some hair but not in appreciable amounts, in some the balding process was retarded and the growth of new hair equalled the loss of old hair, while some had no change at all.

Several factors determined the extent to which minoxidil was successful in these studies. The length of time that balding existed before the use of minoxidil, the less effective the drug was in stimulating new hair growth. The hair on the crown of the head appears to respond to minoxidil better than the hair on the front of the scalp.

Age and general physical health is important, since younger, healthy individuals were more responsive to the medication. Another factor is the type and cause of hair loss; male pattern hair loss appears to be most responsive to minoxidil.

Women who experience male pattern hair loss tend to respond better than men to the regular use of minoxidil.

What is involved in the use of minoxidil?

In the past minoxidil had to be obtained by prescription from a physician, now it is available over the counter at a much more reasonable price.

A dose of 1 milliliter (1/4 teaspoon) of minoxidil is applied to the bald area twice a day at 12-hour intervals for a total daily dose of 2 milliliters (1/2 teaspoon). Exceeding this dose will not necessarily make the hair grow faster nor in greater amounts. It may cause side effects, so it is important to take the recommended dose. Missing an application or two will not interfere with the progress of the treatment unless applications are missed regularly. If an application is missed, the dosage should not be increased to compensate.

Rogaine comes with three different applicators, each of which has a 1 milliliter measurement device. The pump spray tip applicator is used for applying minoxidil to large areas, while the extended spray tip applicator and the rub on applicator are for smaller areas of the scalp.

Minoxidil is absorbed into the scalp in 5 minutes. Because it is odorless and does not leave a residue on the scalp no one but the user needs to know of its use.

It may take up to 3 or 4 months of daily application before results are noticeable. In some cases changes are not obvious for 8 to 12 months. It is necessary to continue the treatment schedule even after hair regrowth is evident in order to maintain the restoration process and to prevent further hair loss. This treatment program is a long term commitment.

If there is no response to the daily use of minoxidil after a

CHAPTER 12

YOUNG AS YOU LOOK

4 month period or more, then it may be worthwhile to consider an alternative.

Does minoxidil cause any side effects?

Though rare, allergic reactions have occurred after the application of minoxidil. An allergic reaction may be characterized by such symptoms as itching, swelling, redness, and a rash. The reactions may be caused by one or more ingredients in the solution, including the minoxidil, alcohol, propylene glycol, and the preservatives.

Problems may also result from the absorption of minoxidil into the body, though this is extremely rare. Hair may grow in areas other than the scalp, and heart problems, such as irregular beating and enlargement of the heart, may occur. Those using minoxidil on a regular basis should be monitored by their physician, even though a prescription is no longer required. If any side effects do occur, use of minoxidil must be discontinued immediately and the physician contacted.

Are there any other agents or medication available for regrowth of hair?

Electric stimulation of the hair follicles has also proven to be a potential hair regrowth solution. Further evaluation of this technique is required before it is made widely available.

Finasteride, when taken orally, is proving effective in stimulating the regrowth of hair in men with male pattern baldness. Originally used to treat benign prostrate enlargement in men, a noted side effect was the regrowth of hair on the scalp. The mechanism of action is the inhibition of the release of an enzyme which transforms testosterone into a potent hormone known as drotestosterone (DHT). DHT stimulates the production of prostate tissue and the shrinkage of hair follicles on the scalp. By restricting the production of DHT, prostate enlargement is reduced and hair follicle growth is allowed to continue along its normal course. It only has an effect on the hair follicles of the scalp, not the rest of the body because it is these hair follicles which are particularly sensitive to shifts and changes in testosterone levels in the body.

Finasteride is already approved by the Food and Drug Administration in the United States as a treatment for benign prostrate enlargement and is currently being evaluated as a medication for baldness. If it is approved as a treatment for male pattern baldness it will be available in a smaller dose under the trade name of Propecia.

Surgical Procedures for Restoring Hair

Hair transplantation is a surgical procedure where the hair from one

CHAPTER 12

area of the scalp is moved to an area of baldness. A more youthful appearance is usually the consequence of a hair transplant and many recipients experience heightened self-esteem and self-confidence. These changes are as enduring as the hair that is transplanted.

How soon can a transplant be performed?

It depends on the patient's attitude toward his receding hair. It is not necessary to wait until complete baldness before having a transplant. It may begin with small transplant areas and as the hair recedes new areas of baldness may be filled in.

The surgeon needs to keep future transplants in mind when planning the removal of hair from the donor area.

What is involved in a hair transplant procedure?

Four surgical techniques are available to restore hair growth to the scalp:

Micro, mini and slit grafts:
These are microscopic grafting techniques which have replaced the once popular punch graft method. The use of smaller grafts produces a more natural transition from thinning or baldness to increased hair growth. The tiny grafts do not give the clumped "doll's head"

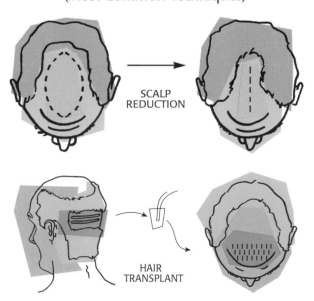

Hair Loss Surgery
(Most Common Techniques)

SCALP REDUCTION

HAIR TRANSPLANT

Donor Site

Recipient Site

appearance after surgery that the punch grafting technique was famous for.

Scalp reduction: A strip of redundant bald skin is removed from the middle of the scalp and the two opposing edges are brought together and stitched. This is particularly useful for the posterior crown of the head where graft procedures are not as successful, and in cases where large areas of baldness limit the amount of donor hair available for grafting methods.

Strip graft: A strip of hair from the back of the head is transplanted into an area of baldness. This technique is commonly used for eyebrow replacement surgery.

Flaps: This procedure is used much less often than other methods. A flap of hair is taken from the side of the head and pivoted over the balding area on top of the head.

Micro, Mini and Slit Grafts

Micro, mini and slit grafts are the most common surgical methods to restore hair growth. The same principles of pre-operative, operative, and post-operative care apply to the other procedures as well. What is cut and where it is placed is what varies.

The following steps are those taken in preparation for a transplant procedure:

■ It is advisable not to drink any alcohol or take medications containing acetylsalicylic acid (aspirin) for 10 days before the surgery, since these substances encourage bleeding. It is also important to inform the surgeon of other medications you might be taking as these could have adverse effects, particularly with respect to bleeding. If indicated, blood tests may be ordered.

■ The hair is allowed to grow at least 3 inches prior to the surgery.

■ The hair is shampooed with regular shampoo the night before or the morning of surgery. Hair spray and other grooming products should not be used once the hair is clean.

The first step is to remove the graft from the donor area, or back and sides of the head:

■ A row of hair at the back of the head is raised, and taped or clipped out of the way. Then the hair to be transplanted is trimmed close to the scalp.

■ The area is anesthetized locally and narrow bands or strips of skin and hair are removed. The density of the hair in the area will determine the number of grafts that the strips will yield. Two strips will usually yield 200 to 300 grafts of 1 to 5 hairs

■ While the donor site is being sutured closed, the strips are cut into mini grafts which are

CHAPTER 12

trimmed and spicules of hair (hairs with no roots) are removed. The grafts are then stored in cool saline while the recipient slits are being prepared on top of the head.

■ The taped hair above the donor site is released to hide the sutures.

■ Once the donor area has been sutured, the recipient area is anesthetized and the slits where the grafts are to be placed are cut. They are approximately 2 to 4 mm long. The recipient slits are generally made in rows following the path of a new hairline.

■ The hair grafts are then rapidly inserted into the slits so the angle of the hair is in a forward position. The degree of the angle is determined by the extent of hair loss, the hairline adjacent to the transplanted area, and the way in which the hair is combed.

■ Gentle pressure is applied to the grafts during surgery and subsequently by a turban-like bandage which covers the donor and the recipient sites and is left in place for 24 hours.

■ The time the total procedure takes varies according to the physician performing the surgery, the number of grafts, and any complications that may arise. As a general rule, it takes about 2 hours.

What care is necessary after the procedure?

Mild discomfort at both the donor and recipient sites may be experienced for 1 to 2 days after the surgery, but can easily be controlled with analgesic medications, such as Tylenol. Once again acetylsalicylic acid (aspirin) should be avoided.

The turban-like bandage is left on overnight and removed the next day by the surgeon, the nursing staff, or by the patient at home. The affected areas are gently cleansed with a sterile solution, such as hydrogen peroxide. Surprisingly little discomfort is felt after the procedure. Painkillers, however, may be prescribed, to be available if needed.

The hair may be combed the day after the procedure, but great care must be taken to avoid accidently hooking and dislodging the grafts. Two days later, the hair can be rinsed and after 3 or 4 days, gently shampooed. Care must be taken not to dislodge the grafts during the first 2 weeks. After this period of time they cannot be pulled out.

The sutures at the donor site are removed after 7 days. After 2 weeks the crusts overlying each graft are carefully removed. Progress is reviewed after 3 months.

What can be expected as time passes?

A small scab forms over each graft. The scabs are sloughed within 1 to 2 weeks and the area is pink for a couple of months.

In the recipient area, the transplanted hair goes into "shock" and falls out within 2 to 8 weeks after the surgery. In about 3 months new hair begins to grow and continues to grow at its normal rate of about half an inch per month.

The donor site gradually heals to a fine white line and is easily camouflaged with the hair in the area.

How long will transplanted hair last?

The transplanted hair will grow for as long as the hair of the donor site from which it has been harvested. In most cases it will last a lifetime.

As time passes most individuals continue to lose their hair. Therefore further transplants are usually required.

Is there a minimum or maximum time period that is allowed between individual sessions?

Minimum time intervals depend on the number of the grafts that can be harvested from the donor site and transplanted to the area of baldness, the extent of the baldness, as well as on each individual's circumstances. The shorter the time interval the more rapidly the hair transplant is completed. Usually sessions are performed at 3 to 4 month intervals if the same area is being transplanted. If different areas are being treated the time interval may be much shorter. There is no maximum interval between sessions.

When there is a large area of baldness, is it possible to cover the entire area?

This is dependent on the size of the donor area. Generally, when there is extensive baldness, a scalp reduction may be performed to decrease the area of baldness to a manageable size. Subsequently, grafting is done to camouflage the scalp reduction scar and to fill in the remaining areas of baldness. The end result may give the appearance of thinned hair rather than absent hair.

What complications are possible?

The incidence of complications is low, and when they do occur are relatively minor.

The scalp is rich with blood vessels and therefore excessive bleeding is possible. It can usually be brought under control with pressure and, if necessary, with sutures. Infection is rare and can be controlled with antibiotics. Problematic scarring is also rare but may occur and depends largely on the patient's predisposition to keloid formation.

Minigrafts & Micrografts

BEFORE

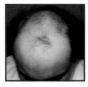

AFTER

PHOTOS COURTESY OF DR. JANICE LIAO (DERMATOLOGIST)

CHAPTER 12

Grafts that refuse to take are an unusual occurrence. More often than not the cause of graft failure is that the grafts are pulled out accidentally or are lost due to scalp injury. An unsatisfactory hairline may be adjusted by inserting more grafts or by removing them.

Hair loss of nontransplanted hair may occur in the recipient area. This is commonly noted in an area of marked thinning. The hair that is lost is hair that is genetically predestined to fall out but the transplant tends to accelerate the attrition rate.

Ingrown hairs or pebbled graft sites may occur. Usually extraction with a needle and time will rectify this situation.

Swelling of the forehead occurs most commonly when larger sections of the front portion of the scalp are transplanted. When the swelling extends to the eyelids black eyes may result. In the 2% of cases that this occurs it is resolved within 4 ro 8 days after the procedure.

Other problems may include allergic reactions to the anesthetic, pigmentary differences between grafts and the recipient areas, and other equally rare complications all easily managed and corrected by the attending surgeon.

Are laser assisted hair transplants superior to scalpel transplants?

Although the use of laser light as a scalpel for hair transplantation is popular, many surgeons would agree that it is not optimal and that the use of a scalpel is still preferable. Although the laser seals the blood vessels as it cuts providing better control over bleeding, the transference of heat to the surrounding tissue tends to discourage the grafts from being accepted at the recipient site. Laser assisted hair transplants are also very operator dependent. Newer developments may eventually make this the methodology of the future, but this is not yet the case.

What do transplants cost and who performs them?

Cost varies with the extent and type of procedure. With the advent of micrografts some surgeons charge their patients on a per session basis ranging from $2,500 to $6,000 each session. The price is sometimes established on a per graft basis. On average, one graft will range in price from $25 to $50. A full transplant may involve between 200 and 800 grafts. It is advisable to discuss this with the surgeon prior to treatment.

Dermatologists and plastic surgeons generally perform transplant surgery.

Treatment for Male Pattern Baldness

	Medication	Surgery	Camouflage
Intervention	• Topical minoxidil (Rogaine, Apogaine, Minoxigaine).	• Hair transplants. • Scalp reductions and grafts.	• Wigs, hair pieces, hair weaving, tunnel, grafting.
Advantages	• Possibility of normal hair. • Low risk.	• Permanent. • Few procedures.	• No surgery or medication.
Disadvantages	• Ongoing expense. • Long-term commitment.	• Costly. • Uncomfortable procedure.	• Temporary. • Artificial. • Ongoing expense.
Potential Problems	• Does not work for everyone. • Allergic reactions, rare. • Heart problems from chemical absorption, rare.	• Scarring, rare. • Infections, rare. • Bleeding, rare.	• Hair wig mismatch, common. • Infection or scarring with tunnel grafting. • Texture mismatch, common. • Incorrect fit. • Frequent adjustments. • Skin irritation under wig.

Camouflaging Hair Loss

Numerous methods exist to camouflage hair loss. Wigs and hair pieces differ immensely in cost, durability, maintenance requirements, and quality. Some are fixed to the skin with glue, others are simply placed on the head, and some are attached to "tunnel grafts", surgically constructed pockets in the skin to which the hairpiece is clipped. Tunnel grafting may cause major problems, including infection and scarring. The skin may be permanently damaged to such an extent that it will no longer be possible to choose alternative methods of regrowing the hair, such as medication or surgery.

Hairpieces should be chosen with care to ensure that the color of the hair matches, the hair has a natural texture and look, and it fits properly. The slightest discrepancy in any of these factors will make the hairpiece noticeable, and an obvious hairpiece looks far worse than a bald head.

Hair weaving is another camouflage option. In this method, hair, usually of human origin, is matched in color and texture to the individual's own hair, then woven or knotted to it. This method works especially well in a small area. The advantage of hair weaving is that it stays in place during vigorous activity, as well as in the water. The disadvantage is that it requires frequent adjustments because as the hair to which it is attached grows, the knots loosen up, and the woven hair lifts away from the head. Irritation of the skin under the woven hair is common, whether or not the hair used is real or synthetic.

The *Breasts*

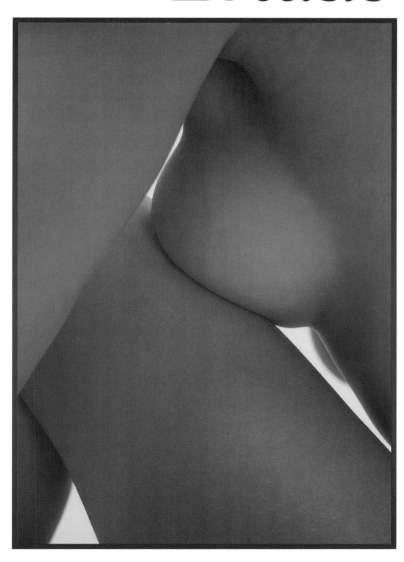

THE SEXUAL FOCUS

A woman's breasts are one of the focal points of sexual attention. Both fashion and society in general combine to dictate the acceptable appearance of the breasts, and, naturally, a large segment of the female population will not be within these norms.

CHAPTER 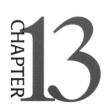13

As with the face, a sense of balance is important with the breasts. With surgery, what nature has done either through time or by accident of birth can be corrected, and the results can be dramatic.

O*ur agenda for a better bust includes:*

▮ *small breasts*
▮ *large breasts*
▮ *breasts that droop*

The development of breasts is one of the first outward signs of transition from girlhood to womanhood. The breasts symbolize sexual attraction and are a means of nurturing children. It is no wonder they are a focal point of attention for both women and men.

The desire for a certain size breast varies with fashion trends. In the late 1920's and 1960's small breasts were in style, whereas from the late 1970's on, larger breasts were fashionable. Now the trend is shifting again.

Women want to alter the shape and size of their breasts for many reasons and should tell their physician what they desire before embarking on surgical procedures. Physicians should clear up any misconceptions about the surgery and its effect on body image and ensure that there are no unrealistic expectations about what the surgery can do.

The reasons for a breast change play an important role in whether or not the outcome will be satisfactory. It is unrealistic to expect a breast change to maintain or establish an interpersonal relationship, obtain a job promotion, save a marriage, or change a lover's behavior. There is no such thing as an emergency breast change. The decision to change the breasts should be well thought out and should be self motivated. Surgery can improve breasts that are too small, too large, or droopy.

SMALL BREASTS

Laura was very self-conscious about her narrow, drooping breasts, so much so that in the early years of her marriage her husband had never seen her naked. A breast enlargement added substantial volume, filled out the excess skin, and raised the nipple slightly. The result was a more attractive, larger breast which improved the way she felt about herself.

Women typically seek breast enlargement to improve their self-image and to look better both in and out of clothing.

Breast Implants

A lack or loss of breast volume may be due to under-development of the breast, a significant amount of weight loss, or pregnancy and breast-feeding. After pregnancy, some women's breasts have less volume and stretched, loose skin. The result is a flat, droopy appearance. This may happen with or without breast-feeding. Breast enlargement is sought to recover the size and posture of the breast prior to pregnancy. As long as the

Cosmetic Surgery of the Breasts

	Augmentation	Reduction	Lift
Description	Enlarging the breast with implants either below or above the muscle tissue to improve breast posture.	Breast tissue and excess skin removed and nipple raised. Visible scar.	Excess skin removed and nipple is raised. No breast tissue removed. Inverted T-scar.
Condition Treated	• Too much breast skin. • Loss of breast volume. • Drooping breasts if the nipple is above the inframammary fold. • Small, underdeveloped breasts. • Breast reconstruction after a mastectomy.	• Excess breast skin. • Excess breast volume. • Large, over-developed breasts. • Functional problems such as backaches.	• Excess breast skin. • Drooping breasts where the nipple hangs below the inframammary fold.
Procedure	• 1 to 1 1/2 hours. • General anesthetic. • Out-patient basis. • Recovery: 1 to 2 weeks.	• 2 to 3 hours. • General anesthetic. • Out-patient basis. • Recovery: 2 to 3 weeks.	• 1 to 1 1/2 hours • Local anesthetic and intravenous sedation • Out-patient basis. • Recovery: 2 to 3 weeks.
Potential Complications (excessive scarring, bleeding and reaction to the anesthetic are rare.)	• Encapsulation of implant with scar: hard breast (5%). • Potential of human adjuvant disease is yet not clear.	• Sensation in nipple lost or altered. • Inability to breast-feed (50%).	• Sensation in nipple lost or altered.
Cost	• $1,500 to $4,000.	• $1,500 to $4,000.	• $1,500 to $4,000.

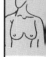

CHAPTER **13**

nipple does not fall below the crease where the breast meets the chest wall (the inframammary crease), a breast enlargement will slightly raise the nipple, fill out the extra skin, and re-establish the lost volume. The actual breast itself remains the same size. The implant simply pushes the existing breast and underlying muscle forward to give the illusion of a larger breast. Women whose breast posture and tone is poor, and whose nipples fall below the inframammary crease, require a breast lift before an enlargement can be done.

Implants are also used to reconstruct the breasts after a mastectomy for cancer. This is important to the self-esteem of many breast cancer victims.

What types of implants are used?

The goals are to create an attractive, symmetrical bust and to produce the desired breast size.

Injections of liquid silicone were used in the early 1950's and proved to be disastrous because of the body's reaction to the silicone fluid. It left many women with lumpy, hard breasts that were often swollen and painful. Silicone injections are never used today.

Fat taken from other parts of the body has been injected into the breasts on an experimental basis, and has proven to be of only temporary benefit. The injected fat gradually decomposes and is replaced by fibrous tissue.

Until recently most physicians used silastic-silicone gel implants, which are made of a silicone gel encased in a bag made of a silicone elastomer. At a molecular level the bag is distinguished from the gel by the amount of cross-linked molecules. The bag has more of these molecules giving it a rubber-like texture. The purpose of the bag is to prevent the silicone gel from coming into contact with the breast tissue, however, it does not provide a complete seal resulting in microscopic leakage. This leaves a slight film of gel on the outer surface of the implant known as a silicone bleed. In the newer generation of implants, the amount of silicone bleed has been significantly reduced by increasing the thickness of the bag. There is some question, however, as to whether the bag itself also sheds silicone into the body over time as it gradually deteriorates.

It has been suggested that the introduction of silicone into the body may play a role in human adjuvant disease (HAD), which is implicated in such conditions as rheumatoid arthritis, systemic lupus erythematosus, dermatomyositis, polymyositis, and perhaps even chronic fatigue syndrome. At present a definitive causal relationship has not been established and the current data would suggest that there is no relationship. However, as with all statistics, the data can be interpreted to either support or refute the claims that silicone contributes to HAD and hence the controversy. For this reason, there is a temporary suspension of the use of the silicone gel implants, until more data is available. In the United States, silicone implants can only be used for breast reconstruction that was planned prior to the moratorium, for the replacement of ruptured implants and in some other very select and carefully monitored situations. In Canada silicone implants have been banned in all circumstances until the controversy has been settled.

So what are the alternatives?

Saline implants are currently the most popular alternative. A saline implant is made of a salt and water solution encased in a bag made of silicone elastomer. These implants are not as popular because they do not look or feel as natural as the silicone gel implants. The saline can also leak through the silastic bag but is not implicated in the HAD controversy because the salt and water are simply absorbed into the body. The only concern with the leak is that the implant may decrease in size over time. The question of the shedding of silicone from the bag remains. Because the amount is so microscopic over a long period of time, the risk is considered to be very low.

However, the situation is being carefully monitored by the medical profession and the regulatory bodies for any adverse effects.

Recently, soybean oil is being used in the silastic bag instead of saline. The advantages of this new alternative is that a woman's breasts have a more natural shape and feel to them.

Where are breast implants placed?

The implant may be placed under the breast tissue (subglandular augmentation mammoplasty) or under the muscle (submuscular augmentation mammoplasty). The submuscular technique involves the insertion of an implant into a pocket created under the muscle over which the breast sits and has been the preferred technique for a number of years. The submuscular technique tends to be more popular because the breasts look and feel more natural, have natural cleavage, and the incidence of subsequent breast hardening is dramatically reduced as compared to the subglandular approach.

The submuscular implant, however, has drawbacks as well. There tends to be more discomfort immediately after the surgery. On contraction of the chest wall muscle (pectoralis major), the implant underneath the muscle is squeezed flat and pushed sideways. Some women find this unattractive. Submuscular implants affect the

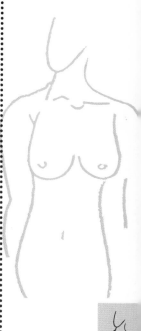

CHAPTER 13

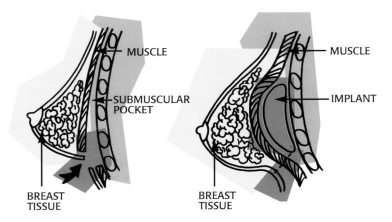

Submuscular Breast Implant

MUSCLE

SUBMUSCULAR POCKET

BREAST TISSUE

MUSCLE

IMPLANT

BREAST TISSUE

performance of such athletes as competitive swimmers and professional weight trainers, who depend on the pectoralis major muscle.

A new technique for inserting the implants has revived the popularity of the subglandular augmentation. The transumbilical breast augmentation (TUBA) technique involves the feeding of the implant up to the breasts through an endoscope which is inserted into an incision in the belly button and fed up to the breasts under the skin. The scar is virtually undetectable and the surgery itself is less invasive than the other techniques. The disadvantage is that accurate placement of the implant may be difficult to achieve.

What is the size of the implant?

Size is determined by the woman's desires and the surgical possibilities. The size of the pocket in which the implant is placed is determined by the size of the breast and chest wall. The implant must fit comfortably into the pocket. An oversized implant is not stuffed into a small pocket and a small implant is not placed into a large pocket. The implant must fit the breast. This will normally create a breast in keeping with the patient's build and chest wall size. Women who request a breast size larger than average will require exceptionally large pockets fashioned under the muscle with subsequent insertion of an oversized implant. The result may not be very attractive.

YOUNG AS YOU LOOK

CHAPTER 13

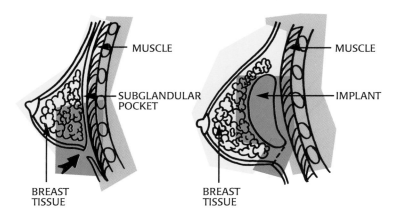

Subglandular Breast Implant

MUSCLE

SUBGLANDULAR POCKET

BREAST TISSUE

MUSCLE

IMPLANT

BREAST TISSUE

What is the procedure for surgery?

■ The incision for breast enlargement may be made in the inframammary fold under the breast where it attaches to the chest wall, around the nipple (known medically as peri-areolar), from the outer edge of the armpit (the transaxillary approach) or directly across the nipple areola. The most common incision is a cut 4 centimeters (1 1/2 inches) in length along the inframammary fold. This makes it easy to create the implant pocket under the muscle, does not disturb the breast tissue too much, and the resulting scar is inconspicuous. The transumbilical (TUBA) technique places the incision in the umbilicus or belly button. The pocket for the implant is created through an endoscope and the silicone bag is put in place. Then saline solution is pumped into the bag to achieve the desired size and shape.

■ Once the implant is in place, the incision is usually closed with absorbable sutures and skin tapes. It is then covered with a light dressing, and a soft elastic bra is placed over the breasts.

■ Some surgeons ask their patients to massage the breasts 3 or 4 times a day during the post-operative period, although this is not usually necessary if an adequate pocket has been made for the implant.

■ After one week most swelling and bruising of the breast has subsided. It is not advisable to purchase a new bra in a larger size for at least 3 weeks after surgery to ensure that all swelling has disappeared. A final check of the breasts is made at 6 weeks.

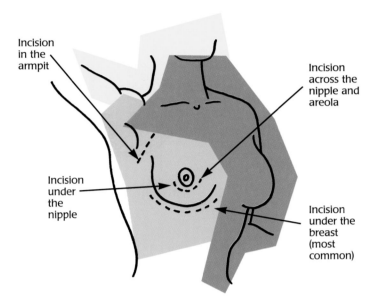

Incision Lines for Breast Augmentation

Incision in the armpit

Incision across the nipple and areola

Incision under the nipple

Incision under the breast (most common)

How long does the surgery take?

Augmentations of both breasts take approximately one hour. The patient returns home with a responsible adult on the day of the surgery. Those with other medical problems, such as asthma and diabetes, are usually kept overnight in the hospital, for closer post-operative monitoring, and discharged the following day.

Does the surgery hurt?

Some discomfort may be experienced over the breast and the front of the armpit for approximately 3 or 4 days. This discomfort gradually

subsides. By the seventh day most discomfort disappears, although occasional shooting pains may be felt in the breast area. This might occur for up to 6 months following surgery, but the frequency gradually decreases as the breasts heal.

Are there any complications with breast augmentations?

All surgery has potential complications. The degree of risk must be weighed with the desired outcome. A breast augmentation can cause the following problems:

■ *Breast Hematoma:*
When blood collects in the implant pocket it is called a

hematoma. One or both breasts swell and marked pain and tightness is felt as well. Any suspicion of a hematoma, even if small, should be investigated by the surgeon. If a hematoma is present, the pocket of the breast is reopened and the blood is drained. As drainage occurs the breast becomes soft again. If a hematoma remains untreated, a capsular contracture that hardens the breast will almost invariably occur.

■ *Capsular Contracture:*
When a layer of fibrous tissue surrounds or encapsulates the implant it is called capsular contracture. Occasionally, excess scar tissue develops around the implant resulting in a hard, often tender breast. This may progress to the point where breast asymmetry occurs, necessitating a second operation through the same incision to remove the fibrous tissue. With the advent of submuscular augmentation, the incidence of capsular contracture has markedly decreased; approximately 1 in 20 women (5%) will develop a firm breast capsule. The exact cause of breast capsular contracture is unknown.

With submuscular breast enlargements, most breasts that are soft at 6 weeks remain that way, although a delayed fibrous contracture may develop in the odd case. This is most likely due to an unrecognized hematoma in one breast causing an increased amount of scarring around one of the implants. To re-establish breast symmetry, surgical correction is necessary.

■ *Decreased Breast Sensation:*
It is common to notice a change or decrease in breast sensation for the first 3 to 6 weeks following surgery. Usually, normal sensation returns. Approximately 1% of women, however, will have a permanent change in nipple sensation. This is usually caused by damage to the nerves of the nipple, which could be due to surgical injury or compression by the implant or scar tissue.

■ *Infection:* This is such a rare complication of breast surgery that most surgeons do not place their patients on pre- or post-operative antibiotics. It is possible that a low-grade infection around the implant is responsible for capsular contractures, but this has not been scientifically confirmed.

Some individuals mistakenly associate the above complications as signs of human adjuvant disease (HAD). This is not the case. These are localized problems related to the surgery and unrelated to the immune system.

CHAPTER 13

Will there be a scar?

There is a scar approximately 4 cm (1 1/2 inches) long in the infra-mammary fold, around the nipple, or in front of the armpit, depending on where the incision was made. The scar in the umbilicus is smaller when the TUBA technique is used. As a general rule, these scars take from 12 to 24 months to heal completely from a red line to a fine white line, but this varies from patient to patient. If the scar is visible, it may be camouflaged cosmetically. Nothing can be placed on the incision (for example, vitamin E) that will speed healing or reduce the size of the scar.

If the scar is problematic and does not heal to a fine white line the appearance may be improved with laser surgery. The type of laser and the technique used will depend on the components of the scar to be treated. If it is red, a vascular laser may be used. A pigment removal laser is used for brown discoloration and a carbon dioxide laser for resurfacing an uneven scar.

How much bigger will the breast be?

Most women increase one or two breast sizes; that is, from a 34A to a 34B or C or from a 36A to a 36B or C. A larger breast may be made, if so desired.

How soon after surgery may activity be resumed?

Normal activity is possible soon after a breast augmentation provided it does not cause discomfort and pain. During the first week after surgery, the patient is aware of the pectoralis muscle. Opening a door by pushing with the shoulder rather than with the arms is probably more comfortable during the first week after surgery. Strenuous activities should be avoided. Patients who do not heed this warning experience much more discomfort and run the risk of developing a hematoma in the implant pocket. A gradual build-up to a full range of activities, such as aerobics, jogging, and swimming, may take place over a 6 week period. The rule of thumb is: if it hurts, do not do it!

Women who lift weights should avoid pectoral curls or other exercises using the pectoral muscles, as this may tear the scar tissue which forms around the pocket after the incision heals. Vigorous stress on these muscles may cause the muscles to tear, resulting in capsular contractures.

A car may be driven the day following surgery, although a standard shift is often uncomfortable to use. There is no restriction on flying.

Is breast-feeding still possible?

Both submuscular and subglandular breast implants are behind the breast tissue, which means they are out of the way of the breast's most important function, that of nurturing a baby. The breast responds to pregnancy induced hormones and enlarges and produces milk. With the increased volume and stretching of the breast during pregnancy, some loss of breast posture may occur, just as it does in the breast which is not augmented.

What happens to the breasts 20 years after surgery?

The implant is medically inert and remains intact far longer than human tissue. The breasts continue to age, with a gradual loss of tone. The scar tissue around the implant, in fact, may actually act as an internal bra, providing some support to the breast.

What can be done about hard and unattractive implants?

Three alternatives may be chosen to solve this problem when a subglandular technique has been used. One is a closed capsulotomy, which is nonsurgical. The breast is compressed from the outside to fracture the scar tissue of the breast capsule. This leaves a softer breast. This solution, however, tends to be temporary because the scar tissue usually redevelops. In some patients, however, the softer breast is maintained.

Another alternative is called open capsulotomy. Here the implant is removed through the incision of the original surgery. The scar tissue that has enclosed or encapsulated the implant is opened and partially removed. The implant

is then reinserted. With subglandular breast augmentation, the incidence of scar tissue recurrence following this procedure is 30 to 40%.

The third alternative is the submuscular implant. The subglandular implant is removed and the original pocket closed. A submuscular pocket is then created, and a larger implant inserted. Although this is the most costly alternative, it is often the best.

Two other, less satisfactory, alternatives would be to accept the deformity and leave the breast untreated or to simply remove the implant (easily done under local anesthetic). Although the stretched skin tends to tighten up over a 6 week period, the breast sags more than it did prior to augmentation.

What happens if encapsulation occurs with a submuscular implant?

It is not possible to treat major encapsulation in a submuscular augmentation without performing surgery. The use of a closed capsulotomy, as in the case of the subglandular implant, does not work because of the deep placement of the implant. If the capsules which develop are really troublesome (hard, tender, asymmetrical breasts), an open capsulotomy is necessary. In this case, the original incision is reopened, and the scar tissue which forms the capsule is

CHAPTER 13

released. The submuscular pocket is enlarged and the implant is then reinserted. Small drainage tubes are often used for the first few days after surgery to ensure that no blood clots collect around the implants.

Do breast implants cause cancer?

Currently, there is no scientific evidence to suggest that the incidence of cancer increases with the introduction of implants into the breasts.

Will it still be possible to detect cancer after an augmentation?

Breast augmentation does not increase or decrease the incidence of breast cancer. In the case of subglandular implants, some breast tissue atrophy and thinning occurs from compression of the implant on the breast substance. This makes detection of masses or cancer on standard mammography difficult, so specialized mammography techniques must be used. With submuscular implants, there is a minimal amount of thinning of the breast tissue. Therefore, concern over cancer detection using standard mammography is less of a problem. Another advantage of submuscular augmentation is that a breast biopsy may be performed without disturbing the implant. With a subglandular augment, the implant is often damaged during a biopsy due to its more superficial location.

Will an augmentation rid the breast of stretch marks?

Stretch marks cannot be eliminated by enlarging the breast, although they often appear less noticeable because the stretch marks are flattened over the larger breast mound.

Will a breast enlargement improve an overweight figure?

Ultimately, the best route to a better figure is to lose any excess weight and to keep it off. Although the breast may be enlarged in overweight women, the result is less attractive because the thick, fatty layer under the skin limits the amount of projection. Much larger implants are necessary to obtain a satisfactory result.

What are the alternatives to surgery?

The only alternative is to wear a padded bra. Exercise will not increase the breast size itself. The muscle beneath the breast will enlarge with certain types of exercises, which, in effect, increases breast projection but not breast size. Any other external techniques to increase the breast size as is advertised in some magazines are a hoax and not valid.

Who performs the surgery and how much does it cost?

Board certified cosmetic surgeons usually with a background in

YOUNG AS YOU LOOK

plastic surgery who are trained in the techniques discussed perform breast augmentations. The costs range anywhere from $1,500 to $4,000.

LARGE BREASTS

Contrary to some people's belief, large breasts are not a godsend. They frequently cause functional problems with neck, shoulder, and back discomfort and poor posture, breast pain and heaviness, breathing difficulties due to breast weight, deep shoulder grooves, and moisture and skin rashes under and between the breasts. Large, pendulous breasts are often unattractive because gravity causes them to lose their shape and the nipples are lowered. It is also difficult to find clothes and bras that fit and to enjoy physical activity. Beyond these physical problems, psychological stress may be suffered, due to the attention large breasts attract.

Breast Reductions

Women who undergo breast reductions are among the happiest with the results of their surgery. Imagine how removing 2 to 3 pounds or more from the chest improves the posture and appearance and creates a better self-image.

Most cases of oversized breasts (80%, in fact) develop during puberty. The other 20% occur after pregnancy, menopause, or following substantial weight gain.

A breast reduction can reduce the breast volume, raise the nipples to the correct height, reshape the breast to produce an esthetically pleasing breast posture, and correct gross asymmetry.

What is involved in breast reduction?

A variety of techniques are available to reduce breast size. The specific technique varies from surgeon to surgeon and depends on breast size and shape, the patient's age and associated medical problems, and the results desired. The essential steps are as follows:

■ Prior to surgery, a photograph of the breasts is taken. The planned incisions are drawn on the breasts while the patient is in a sitting position. A general anesthetic is then administered.

■ A keyhole incision is made around the nipple and down to the inframammary fold. With most techniques the incision extends along the inframammary fold to leave an inverted "T" shaped scar pattern. The nipple-areolar complex and its underlying breast tissue with the accompanying blood supply and nerves are preserved in order to maintain sensation and circulation to the nipple.

Breast Reduction

BEFORE

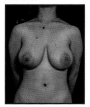

AFTER

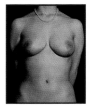

PHOTOS
COURTESY OF
THE CANADIAN SOCIETY
FOR AESTHETIC (COSMETIC)
PLASTIC SURGERY

CHAPTER 13

Closure Lines for Breast Reductions and Lifts

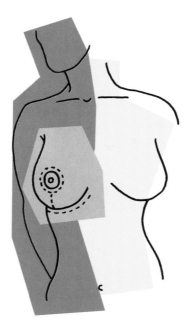

A more recent technique developed by Dr. M. Lejour avoids the scar under the breast. The incision extends from around the nipple-areolar complex down to the inframammary fold but not along the fold. This procedure is best used for reduction of smaller breasts.

- Excess breast tissue and skin within the incisions is then removed and in some cases fat is sucked out using a lipo-suction technique. The nipple-areolar complex is raised to the planned height, and the incisions are closed.

- Approximately 50% of women can still breast-feed when this technique is used. For women with very large breasts, or for those who are older and have medical problems, the nipple and areolar complex is often totally removed and reapplied using a grafting technique. In this case, there is little or no residual sensation in the nipple and breast-feeding is not possible.

- Drainage tubes are usually inserted into both breasts. This enables any accumulated fluid or blood to drain into the dressing. The drainage tubes are removed and the dressings changed 48 hours after surgery. Normally, the incisions heal within two weeks, and no further dressings are necessary. Women who smoke, however, tend to heal more slowly, particularly at the juncture of the inverted "T". This is due to the constriction of the small blood vessels within the skin caused by the nicotine, as well as a reduced blood supply caused by the incision and the tension exerted upon the breast skin at the point of closure. Women are cautioned not to smoke for ideally 5 months but minimally 2 days prior to surgery and a week or 2 following surgery.

- In most cases swelling and bruising from the surgery is resolved by the tenth to fourteenth day, at which time the sutures are removed. If the sutures are absorbable, this is not necessary. The patient is advised not to shop for a new bra for approximately 3 to 4 weeks following surgery to allow swelling to completely subside. Occasionally, some leakage is noted along the incision from the previous drainage tube sites. This subsides as the bruising and swelling disappear.

How much breast tissue is removed?

The amount of breast tissue to be removed is determined prior to surgery by both the woman and her surgeon. It is essential that the surgeon understands what the expectations are in order to avoid dissatisfaction with the results. Some women desire that only a small amount of the breast volume be removed, their main concern being the restoration of breast tone and shape. Other individuals prefer much smaller breasts.

Will there be a scar?

Any surgical procedure that involves the cutting of tissue leaves a scar. The way the incision heals and the scar forms is genetically determined. Therefore, some women end up with fine, barely visible white lines, whereas others have more obvious scars. Normally, however, the scars fade to white lines which look similar to stretch marks within 12 to 18 months.

What are the possible complications?

The following are the potential problems that may occur after breast reduction:

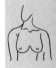

- *Scarring:* Troublesome scars can be cosmetically improved by injecting cortisone into the scar to flatten it, using the vascular lasers to remove residual redness, the pigment removal lasers to treat hyperpigmentation and the carbon dioxide laser to resurface uneven lumps and bumps. If the scar is dramatically white or the nipple has an abnormal appearance color can be implanted into the tissue using medical tattooing techniques.

■ *Hematoma:* A hematoma is a collection of blood. A sudden increase in swelling, pain, and tightness in one or both breasts is an indication that there is a hematoma within the breast. The drainage tubes put in place after surgery remove small amounts of blood and serum but do not prevent hematomas; they must be surgically drained. It is important to realize that hematomas are a potential complication of most types of surgery and are not a reflection of the quality of the surgery. Rather, the early recognition and appropriate treatment of the hematoma is an indication of a surgeon's skill.

■ *Nipple Complications:* Loss of sensation in the nipple is rare and unpredictable. Women with large breasts often have poorer sensation in the nipple area than do women with smaller breasts. Therefore, the potential sensory loss in women requesting a reduction mammoplasty does not seem to be as critical as for women requesting breast augmentations.

The inability to breast-feed is a potential problem as well, and occurs in approximately 50% of cases. There is also a risk, although rare, that the nipple

and areolar complex will die due to an insufficient blood supply following the removal of adjacent breast tissue. This occurs more often in older women, smokers, and women who have diseases such as diabetes or high blood pressure than in other people. This condition is usually recognized at the time of surgery because the nipple and areolar complex turns white or dark blue indicating circulation problems. When this occurs during the operation, the nipple and areolar complex is usually removed and placed on as a graft. If the problem arises after surgery is complete, the nipple and areolar complex, along with the underlying tissue, will die, and the healing process will be prolonged. Over a period of 3 months the dead tissue is removed by the surgeon, while the breast slowly heals. When the site has completely healed, a nipple reconstruction may be considered. Permanent coloration (medical tattooing) of the areola can be helpful in creating a natural appearance of the nipple, in these cases.

■ *Fat Necrosis:* An area of fat that has died as a result of poor blood supply is called fat necrosis. It is characterized by a firm, hard lump in the breast and often some redness of the overlying skin. The body temperature usually increases

CHAPTER 13

224 *YOUNG AS YOU LOOK*

for a few days mimicking an infection. If the necrosis is small, it usually resolves spontaneously over a period of weeks. If the affected area is larger it may require surgical removal of the dead fat, which could result in size asymmetry when healing is complete.

■ *Infection:* Infection rarely occurs in breast reductions and, therefore, antibiotics are not usually prescribed as a precautionary measure after surgery.

What constitutes a poor result in surgery?

The outcome of breast reduction may be unsatisfactory for the following reasons:

■ *Breast Asymmetry:* Most women have some degree of natural breast asymmetry, and exact symmetry following breast reduction is difficult to achieve. If gross asymmetry occurs following surgery, some revisional surgery will likely be necessary.

■ *Poor Nipple Position:* The nipple position is established while the patient is in a sitting position. The position is usually correlated with chest size and overall body height. If the nipple is positioned slightly lower than normal, it can always be raised to a higher position, if necessary. If the nipple is positioned too

high, it is difficult to correct and invariably results in additional scarring on the breast.

■ *Inadequate Breast Reduction:* If enough of the breast has not been reduced, it may be due to a lack of communication between surgeon and patient. Revisional surgery with further reduction is easily performed. Too much reduction of the breast is rare and can only be corrected with a breast augmentation.

■ *Skin Puckers:* The breast ends at the inframammary fold in the region where the arm normally touches the chest wall. In some overweight women, there is considerable fat in this area, which becomes more prominent after the breast is reduced thus causing a skin pucker. The excess fat may be reduced by losing weight or by liposuction after the breast reduction.

How long does the procedure take?

The procedure usually takes 2 to 3 hours, and an overnight stay in the hospital is to be expected. Some medical centers perform the surgery on an outpatient basis.

Does it hurt?

Breasts do not have many nerves, so most discomfort is experienced at the incisions. Moderate discomfort for the first few days after surgery is normal, and painkillers are provided. The discomfort gradually subsides as bruising and swelling decrease.

How soon after surgery can normal activity be resumed?

A normal level of activity can be resumed within one week, depending on the discomfort. Normally, a return to work is possible after 1 to 2 weeks. Heavy lifting or any activity that causes discomfort should be avoided for 6 weeks. As the discomfort subsides, the level of activity may be increased.

If it is comfortable to do so, driving or flying within the first week should not be a problem.

At what age should a breast reduction be performed?

Breast reductions can be performed in girls as young as 12 (who may have a condition known as massive gigantomastia). Women in their sixties and seventies also are candidates.

It is irresponsible to expect a young girl to live with very large breasts,simply because further breast growth may occur following any surgery. As a general rule, if the breasts are excessively large, the surgery is performed even though full maturation has not been reached, with the provision that further breast reduction may be required as the breast grows. A repeat procedure can be done through the same series of incisions

with no added risk.

What about breast cancer or fibrocystic disease?

The risk of developing breast cancer is the same after a breast reduction as before the surgery. But breast reduction surgery changes the appearance of the breast on mammography. Therefore, if fibrocystic disease is being followed by serial mammography, a repeat mammogram will be required 6 months after a reduction to establish a new baseline.

Will a breast reduction get rid of stretch marks?

Stretch marks on the skin that was surgically removed will be gone. The remaining stretch marks are flattened out because the skin over the breasts has been tightened. This makes them less obvious but does not eliminate them.

Will the breasts become smaller with weight loss?

If breasts of normal size become quite large with weight gain, weight loss significantly reduces their volume. As a general rule, though, most women with marked breast enlargement due to weight gain report that their breasts were always large even when they were slimmer. In these women weight reduction has a minimal effect on the overall breast size.

Who performs the surgery and what does it cost?

Board certified esthetic surgeons with a specialization in plastic surgery usually perform this surgery. Prices vary between $1,500 and $6,000, the cost being dependent on the extent of the problem, where the surgery is done, and the surgeon.

BREASTS THAT DROOP

When breast volume and tone are lost, the breast becomes droopy and unattractive. The upper part of the breast is flattened in a pancake-like fashion and the nipple and areolar complex droop below the inframammary crease, frequently pointing to the floor. There is, as well, an excess amount of skin, often marked with striae.

Droopy breasts may occur in young girls if the breast substance is poorly developed and in women who have undergone weight loss, pregnancy, or breast-feeding. This may be further exacerbated by the natural aging process and the pull of gravity. In fact, these last two factors alone may be the cause of droopy breasts.

Breast Lifts

What is involved in a breast lift?

A breast lift (or mastopexy) removes excess skin, raises the nipple to the correct height,

and re-establishes the support of the breast for a more esthetic posture. To provide the necessary volume, a breast lift may be combined with an augmentation.

A breast lift restores the breasts to a more youthful look. The result is a symmetrical, naturally proportioned and positioned breast of appropriate size, shape, and position. A breast lift, however, does not prevent the breasts from aging; they continue to be affected by the pull of gravity and the intrinsic changes that take place with age. Some of the benefits of the breast lift, therefore, are lost over time. Those patients with good skin quality, that is, elastic and flexible skin with minimal or no stretch marks, have a longer lasting result because the skin itself offers better support to the breast tissue.

If droopy breasts are due to weight loss, a breast lift should not be performed until the weight is stable, since further weight loss after surgery may cause a recurrence of the problem. Women who are overweight, with heavy, droopy breasts, often require a breast reduction rather than a breast lift. The pull of gravity on the heavy breast causes a recurrence of the sagging unless some excess tissue is removed.

What is the procedure for surgery?

■ If the procedure involves only a breast lift, it is often performed on an outpatient basis under a local anesthetic with accompanying intravenous sedation. If, however, it is combined with augmentation to increase the breast volume, the procedure is performed under a general anesthetic.

- The keyhole incision used for breast reductions is also used for breast lifts. After excess skin is removed from the keyhole, the nipple and areolar complex are then raised to the planned height. Since the blood and nerve supply to the nipple is not touched in a breast lift, there is no risk of loss of sensation to the nipple and areolar complex. The incision is then closed, leaving an inverted-T closure, and a dressing is applied.

- If augmentation is combined with a breast lift, the implant is put in place prior to removing excess skin to ensure that an adequate amount of skin is available to close the incision. Also, when the skin is draped over the implant it makes the removal of excess skin easier.

- Dressings and stitches are removed within 2 weeks, unless the stitches are self absorbing. Bruising and swelling in a breast lift are not as severe as with a reduction.

- One to 1 1/2 hours is the time usually required to complete a breast lift. If a local anesthetic is used, the patient may return home shortly after the surgery is finished.

Will there be a scar?

A scar is unavoidable. Initially, it is red and thick but, over a year, this gradually fades to a white line, not unlike a stretch mark. The breast lift incision scar resembles the breast reduction scar, but is usually shorter.

Troublesome scars are treated with lasers to smooth lumpiness by resurfacing or remove red or brown discoloration. Medical tattooing can reintroduce pigment into scars which are noticeably devoid of color.

Does it hurt?

The discomfort is mild to moderate and gradually decreases during the first week as swelling and bruising subside.

What are the possible complications?

Infection is possible but rarely occurs. The incision may not heal well, and too much tension in the incision could cause it to separate resulting in a more pronounced scar. Smoking should be avoided during healing as it impedes the blood supply to the incision.

How soon can normal activities be resumed?

Normal activity can be resumed within 3 days and is limited only by the amount of discomfort

YOUNG AS YOU LOOK

experienced. By 6 weeks, healing should be complete. There is no restriction on driving or flying.

Does a breast lift increase the chances of getting cancer?

The risk of developing breast cancer does not increase with this procedure. Patients who are having serial mammographies due to fibrocystic disease are encouraged to have a repeat mammogram at about 6 months to establish a new baseline for their breasts.

Is breast-feeding possible after a breast lift?

The ability to breast-feed remains the same following a breast lift as before. Women should not have a breast lift until they have finished having children because pregnancy and breast-feeding will stimulate a temporary enlargement and stretching of the breast. This may cause further drooping of the breasts, and will counteract the positive benefits of the surgery.

Why might the procedure be unsatisfactory?

If the breasts droop again, it may be due to poor skin quality (lost elasticity and resilience), or heavy breasts. In the case of heavy breasts, the excess breast tissue drops into the lower half of the breast, giving the nipple-areolar complex the appearance of being too high. This can be corrected with a breast reduction where the excess breast tissue is removed from the lower half of the breast. Another reason for sagging breasts could be weight loss after a breast lift. If the problem is due to an inadequate amount of lift or if the breasts are asymmetrical, the procedure can be repeated approximately 12 months after the original surgery using the same incisions.

Who does a breast lift and what is the cost?

A board certified cosmetic surgeon usually with a specialization in plastic surgery performs breast lifts. It costs about $1,500 to $4,000 for a breast lift alone and $2,500 to $6,000 for a breast lift combined with a breast enlargement.

OTHER BREAST PROBLEMS

Breast Asymmetry

A certain degree of breast asymmetry, where one breast is larger than the other, is normal and to be expected. If, however, one breast varies significantly from the other in volume or posture resulting in marked asymmetry, the problem can be corrected using the principles of breast augmentation, reduction, and lift. For example, one breast can be reduced and the other lifted, or one breast can be reduced and the other augmented, or any combination appropriate to correct the asymmetry. These procedures are done

CHAPTER 13

simultaneously or in stages, depending on what is required.

Inverted Nipples

Inverted nipples are fairly common. They are usually inherited and may occur in both nipples or on one side only. In most instances, the ducts leading from the breast to the nipple are underdeveloped, which creates a tethering effect on the nipple preventing its normal protrusion. Most women who have inverted nipples have difficulty breast-feeding.

The surgical procedure to correct this problem is simple and done under local anesthetic. It essentially involves a release of the tethered ducts and the pro-vision of local tissue to support the area beneath the nipple. This is done through a small incision in the areola. Since the ducts connect-ing the breast to the nipple are cut, breast-feeding is no longer possible. Sensation to the nipple remains intact.

Skin Tags

Small tags of excess skin are frequently found under the breasts,

but they may also occur in the armpit, on the neck, and in the groin creases. They may become irritated by clothing, particularly by a bra or by heavy breasts. Small skin tags can be removed without anesthetic by clipping them with a pair of surgical scissors. Large ones may require a local anesthetic. Cryotherapy, electrocauterization, tying off with stitches, and vaporization with a laser are all alternatives for their removal. Avoiding excessive weight gain and constrictive clothing helps prevent skin tags from recurring.

Cherry Angiomas

Cherry angiomas are benign blood vessel tumors that may appear on the breasts as well as on other areas of the torso. They are cosmetically undesirable to many and can be removed easily. The best alternative for removal is the use of a vascular laser such as the variable pulse width (VPW) or the pulse dye laser. Another alternative is electrodesic-cation where the angioma is gently burned away with an electric needle or it is possible to vaporize them with a carbon dioxide laser. These procedures involve minimal to moderate discomfort that is short-lived. Scarring is extremely rare.

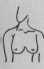

The
Abdomen

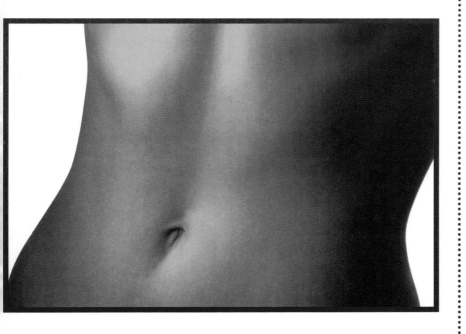

FIRM &
FLATTERING

*Ah, for the
way you
looked when
you were 18!
But time,
pregnancy,
and just too
much of the
good life and
too little
exercise
have taken
their toll.*

Our agenda for a firmer, flatter tummy includes:

■ *abdominal liposuction*
■ *the tummy tuck*

The Rubens look is out and the bikini look is in. Male and female models, with their sleek, smooth abdomens and their next-to-nothing garments have set the trend. The person whose physique is in extreme contrast to the fashion ideal often feels stressed about their looks.

Without a doubt, diet and exercise play an important role in correcting the problem of an oversized abdomen. For most men this is the best solution, but for women the situation is different, and pregnancy is one of the culprits. The skin is stretched to its limit leaving many women with redundant skin and stretch marks. Muscle tone is lost and persistent fat deposits are a problem.

So what can be done? A lifestyle shift to include regular physical activities and a well balanced diet should be the first step. Help is available through weight loss and fitness centers. When the weight and fitness level that one can comfortably maintain is reached, the help of an esthetic surgeon may be sought.

The recommended cosmetic procedure will depend on the specific problem to be solved. For example, if the skin is sufficiently resilient and elastic with a minimum amount of excess skin, but with too much subcutaneous abdominal fat, abdominal liposuction would be the procedure of choice. On the other hand excess skin and fat, stretch marks, and loss of muscle tone requires a "tummy tuck" or abdominal lipectomy to produce a firm, relatively flat abdomen.

ABDOMINAL LIPOSUCTION

Liposuction is discussed in detail in the *Chapter 15: The Buttocks and Limbs,* including the pros and cons of the tumescent technique versus the dry technique. Here we have presented a brief synopsis of tumescent liposuction of the abdomen.

Liposuction of the abdomen may be performed alone in those with too much subcutaneous abdominal fat if their skin elasticity and muscle tone are good or it may be combined with a tummy tuck. The decision is one of personal choice. For example, a patient who has a bulky tummy which interrupts the natural draping of her clothes may not be too concerned about whether or not the skin is smooth and wrinkle free. Her main concern may simply be the deposits of abdominal fat. In this case liposuction may be adequate to meet her needs. It would certainly be less traumatic.

On the other hand if she wished to achieve a tighter, smoother, flat abdomen, then liposuction in combination with a tummy tuck would be in order.

How is tumescent liposuction of the abdomen performed?

- Tumescent liposuction does not require a general anesthetic. A saline solution which contains a local anesthetic is introduced into the targeted fat deposits. This numbs the area to be treated.

- The incisions are very tiny and are located in strategic positions over the abdomen. A tumescent solution is then injected into the targeted layer of fat. This solution contains saline to prevent dehydration, a local anesthetic to numb the area, a medication to control bleeding and cortisone to control inflammation. Once the area is firm and numb the surgeon begins to remove the fat.

- A very small suction cannula is inserted through the incisions into the tumescent fatty layer of the abdomen. Using a back and forth action the surgeon criss-crosses the abdomen creating a number of tunnels in the fat with a cannula. The cannula is attached to a suction apparatus which draws the fat out from under the skin as the tunnels are created. The number of tunnels created determines the amount of fat that can be removed.

- After an acceptable abdominal contour has been achieved, the incisions sites are covered with absorbent pads and held in place with a pressure garment. Some physicians use a second garment over the first to provide additional pressure. The incisions are not sutured in order that the remaining solution will drain off into the pads. This helps to minimize swelling, bruising, and soreness. Eighty percent of the solution is absorbed into the body and excreted in the urine. The remaining 20% is either sucked out with the fat or drained out through the tiny incisions.

- The pressure garment is worn for a minimum of 4 days. Wearing the garment longer than this tends to decrease swelling sooner but does not alter the ultimate outcome of the procedure.

Does tumescent liposuction of the abdomen hurt?

The anesthetic in the tumescent solution numbs the area to be treated so little or no pain is felt during the procedure. No general anesthetic nor hospital stay is necessary.

Due to the residual local anesthetic and the mild cortisone left in the tissue, most patients do not experience any significant soreness for 6 to 18 hours after the

bar

b

CHAPTER 14

Abdomen Liposuction

BEFORE

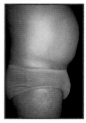

AFTER

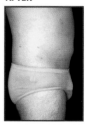

PHOTOS
COURTESY OF
DR. DON GROOT

procedure. An aching sensation similar to that felt in the muscles after rigorous exercises may be experienced for up to 5 days after the surgery. Analgesia, such as Tylenol, helps to control this temporary discomfort.

What will I experience after tumescent liposuction?

Swelling, inflammation and soreness are to be expected. The more fat that has been removed the longer the duration of post-operative swelling and discomfort.

Temporary subcutaneous lumpiness and firmness are also common in the healing process. This may persist to some degree for 2 to 6 months.

Bruising is usually minimal with the tumescent technique because the bleeding is minimized by medication called epinephrine in the saline solution. Any bruising that may occur tends to subside over a period of 10 to 15 days.

When will an improvement be noticed?

About 90% of patients can actually see at least some improvement in their silhouette one week after surgery. However, because of the slow resolution of post surgical swelling, the ultimate results following tumescent liposuction is achieved in 12 to 24 weeks.

What are the limitations and alternatives to liposuction?

Liposuction is not a means to lose or control weight. It is a procedure designed to remove deposits of localized fat which are resistant to diet and exercise. A patient's weight should be stable for 6 months prior to the procedure. Further weight loss after the procedure will only enhance the results. A regular exercise plan will tone the underlying muscles and improve the results of the surgical contouring.

Liposuction is a technique which is used to remove subcutaneous fat (fat under the skin). Many men and women have fat in their abdominal cavity as well as under their skin. Only the fat under the skin can be removed with liposuction. The remaining fat must be lost through diet and exercise.

It is also important for a woman to understand that removing subcutaneous fat from the belly may not lead to a flat abdomen, especially if the abdominal musculature is round. A regular regime of exercises to strengthen the abdominal muscles will be necessary to achieve a flat abdomen. There may be some irregularity if scars, herniations or muscular separation are present.

The only alternative to

CHAPTER 14

Cosmetic Surgery of the Abdomen

	Liposuction	Tummy Tuck
Description	• Excess fat is removed from the abdomen by sucking it out through a tube called a cannula. • Candidates should have good skin elasticity and good muscle tone. • Bruising and swelling after the procedure (much less with the newer tumescent technique).	• A procedure to remove excess skin and fat in lower abdomen and tighten muscles. • Procedure causes considerable discomfort.
Condition Treated	• Excess subcutaneous abdominal fat.	• Excess abdominal skin. • Excess subcutaneous abdominal fat. • Loss of muscle tone.
Procedure	• Time varies depending on the amount of fat to be removed. • A general anesthetic is required with the dry technique but not with the tumescent technique. • Can be done on an out patient basis. • Recovery time: 2 to 6 weeks with the dry technique and 2 to 7 days with the tumescent technique.	• Takes 1 to 1 1/2 hours. • A general anesthetic is required. • Can be done on an out patient basis. • Recovery time: 3 to 4 weeks.
Complications	• Waves, dents or dimples in the skin.	• Temporary sensory loss in abdomen. • Poorly positioned belly button.
Cost	• $2,500 to $6,000.	• $1,500 to $6,000.

abdominal liposuction is extensive dieting. Most people who have decided to have liposuction have been through several dieting programs and have failed to lose their abdominal fat.

CHAPTER 14

THE TUMMY TUCK

Tummy tucks can improve the look of an abdomen which has loose skin with stretch marks (a crumpled looking tummy), and a loss of muscle tone in the lower and upper portion. To a certain extent excess fat is also removed. Women more commonly seek this type of assistance than men. Women who plan to have children are advised against this procedure, since pregnancy stretches the skin and muscle. Slender women with a history of anorexia and bulimia are considered poor candidates due to unrealistic expectations and psychological instability.

What is involved in a tummy tuck?

The tummy tuck is a procedure designed to remove excess skin and fat in the lower portion of the abdomen (from the belly button to the pubic hairline and from hipbone to hipbone) as well as to tighten up the muscles.

■ Prior to surgery a photograph is taken. It provides an accurate record of the problem, and will demonstrate the improvement accomplished with surgery.

■ The plan for surgery is then drawn on the abdomen while the patient is standing. This is necessary since the skin falls differently while standing than sitting. Due to the fact that the surgery is performed with the patient lying down, the map for surgery is essential to help ensure proportionally correct results.

■ A tummy tuck is performed under a general anesthetic and takes approximately 1 1/2 to 2 hours, either on an outpatient basis or with an overnight stay in the hospital. This depends on the patient and the surgeon.

■ The incision for a tummy tuck extends just over the pubic hairline from hipbone to hipbone in a flattened W-shape. A key-hole incision is then made up the center of the lower abdomen and around the belly button.

■ The belly button is left intact, but excess skin and fat from the lower part of the abdomen (from the pubic hairline to the umbilicus and from hipbone to hipbone) is removed.

■ The exposed underlying muscle is tightened.

■ The abdominal skin above the belly button is released from its fibrous attachments and is stretched downward to the pubic hairline.

■ A small incision is made in this new skin cover for the belly button.

■ The large incision is closed so that the scar is within the bikini line.

CHAPTER 14

- Two small openings are left for drainage tubes. These allow any accumulation of fluid or blood to drain into the dressing. The dressings are changed and the tubes removed 48 hours after the procedure.

- Incisions usually heal in two weeks and no further dressings are necessary. The sutures are removed in 10 to 14 days unless they are self-absorbing. Smokers tend to heal more slowly than nonsmokers because smoking inhibits the blood supply to the wound.

- The patient is instructed to wear a girdle or corset over the entire abdominal area to provide support and comfort while healing. This decreases the chance of a seroma (pocket of fluid) from developing.

Will there be swelling and bruising?

Swelling and bruising are inevitable and will subside in 10 to 14 days.

Does it hurt?

This is one of the most uncomfortable cosmetic procedures. Due to the amount of skin removed and the tightening of the muscle, it often takes 1 to 2 weeks before the patient can stand. Full recovery takes at least two weeks. Oral painkillers are prescribed to help control the discomfort. Products containing acetylsalicylic acid (aspirin) are not recommended, as they encourage bleeding.

Some patients experience a burning sensation or tingling over the thighs which gradually subsides within 3 to 4 weeks.

Will a scar be visible?

A scar is unavoidable. It extends from hipbone to hipbone in a flattened W-shape within the bikini line. At first it is quite red and itchy, but eventually turns pink, then fades to a white line. This may take anywhere from 1 to 2 years.

When can normal activities be resumed?

Normal activities should not be resumed for at least two weeks. Assistance at home with young children and normal household duties should be arranged prior to the surgery. Heavy lifting, strenuous exercise, or any activity which causes discomfort should be avoided until 6 weeks after surgery. As the discomfort subsides, the level of activity may gradually be increased.

Should weight be lost before and after the surgery?

Ideally, a person's weight should be stable and at a level which can easily be maintained without extensive dieting.

The same level of fitness and weight established before surgery needs to be maintained after

CHAPTER 14

surgery or the results will be less than optimal. Losing weight after a tummy tuck improves the surgical result and the overall contour of the torso. Gaining weight after surgery causes the problem to recur, and a lower abdominal paunch may develop. This is because excess abdominal skin and fat will hang over the abdominal scar, which acts like a tight belt.

Will stretch marks disappear?

No procedure can remove stretch marks over the entire abdomen. A tummy tuck will remove skin on the lower abdomen thus eliminating stretch marks in this area. The stretch marks on the skin of the upper abdomen which is pulled down to cover the lower abdomen will remain, but will look better because the skin has been stretched.

Regular applications of creams containing tretinoin or the use of laser therapy may help to soften the look of unsightly stretchmarks. These alternatives are discussed in more detail in Chapter 15.

Does a tummy tuck affect the internal organs?

A tummy tuck does not enter the abdominal cavity, and therefore has absolutely no effect on the function of the bowel or other internal organs. Occasionally, a small abdominal wall hernia is discovered during the tummy tuck procedure, and is repaired at the same time.

Can a tummy tuck be combined with a hysterectomy or tubal ligation?

It is theoretically possible to combine these gynaecological procedures with tummy tuck surgery, although the risk of infection and other complications is significantly increased because the abdominal cavity, where the internal organs are located, is entered. There is always some degree of contamination by bacteria when the abdominal cavity is opened. Combining a gynecological procedure with a tummy tuck takes more time and puts the patient at greater risk of developing otherwise rare complications. Therefore, it is usually recommended that simultaneous surgical intervention which would increase the risk to the patient be avoided.

What complications could occur?

A variety of potential complications are associated with the tummy tuck.

■ *Sensory Loss:* Sensory loss over the lower part of the abdomen is common. Generally, 3 to 4 months are required before feeling in this area returns to normal, but the problem may persist for up to a year or two after surgery. Occasionally, a loss of sensation may be felt over the front of the thighs, but this eventually returns.

CHAPTER 14

- **Poorly Positioned Belly Button:** Occasionally, the belly button may be placed too high, too low, or off to the side. This is usually due to an error in surgical judgement. Fortunately, it can easily be relocated with a minor procedure under local anesthetic.

- **Hematoma:** Blood may collect under the skin of the abdomen, and is characterized by a sudden increase in swelling, pain, and tightness of the area. The drainage tubes which are put in place after surgery are used primarily to relieve small collections of blood or fluid. Large hematomas must be surgically drained.

- **Seroma:** A persistent accumulation of fluid underneath the lower abdomen called a seroma may develop. In most instances, the seroma gradually subsides on its own, although in some cases surgical drainage may be required.

- **Contour Irregularities:** Small puckers of bulging skin may occur on the hip side of the incisions. The obese are more prone to this problem because excess skin and fat have been removed from the abdomen, but nothing has been done to the hips. This is easily remedied with liposuction to feather, sculpt, and contour the area, eliminating these irregularities.

- **Skin Slough:** The skin which was stretched over the lower abdomen may, in rare cases, die due to an inadequate blood supply. This occurs most frequently in smokers and in people who are older, obese, or have other medical problems, such as diabetes and high blood pressure. An untreated hematoma or an infection can also cause skin sloughing. When this happens, the dead tissue is removed and the area is allowed to heal, although the healing process often takes up to 3 months and leaves an unsightly scar. A scar revision procedure is often necessary once healing is complete.

- **Infections:** Infections rarely occur, but, when they do, they are usually managed with antibiotics. Surgical drainage is rarely required.

- **Scars:** Scars usually fade to a white line and in women are hidden by most bikinis. If excessive scarring occurs, it can be flattened with a laser or injected with cortisone to make it less obvious. Given enough time, these scars eventually fade.

Who performs the surgery and how much does it cost?

Dermatologists and plastic surgeons trained in tumescent liposuction are qualified to perform the procedure. Tummy tucks are usually performed

CHAPTER 14

by plastic surgeons. The cost varies from $2,000 to $6,000, depending on whether the tummy tuck and liposuction are done alone or in combination.

Special Case: Obese people who have a large apron of abdominal fat and skin may experience abdominal pain and skin problems from stretching and traction of this fatty apron that hangs down over the pubic hair and sometimes onto the thighs. In these patients, the procedure to remove this fatty apron may be diagnosed as a functional and reconstructive problem and may, therefore, be covered by some insurance plans.

The *Buttocks & Limbs*

SYMBOLS OF YOUTH

The buttocks, legs, and arms are symbols of youth. Buttocks are sexually attractive to both men and women, and arms and legs provide sure signs of a person's conditioning.

Our agenda for your buttocks and limbs includes:

■ *fat pads*
■ *cellulite*
■ *stretch marks*
■ *leg veins*
■ *aging hands and feet*

Studies have shown that if a woman's waist to hip ratio is .70 or less men are subconsciously attracted to them. It is assumed that this attraction is tacit and rooted in natural selection because these women are the best candidates for child bearing. However, not all women are blessed with these subliminally seductive proportions and even if they are they tend to change with age.

The buttocks, legs, and arms reflect our agility and youth. Women's legs, for example, are considered to be objects of sexual attraction, particularly as hemlines rise. The weight, color, and tone of the limbs change with age, and people become concerned about contour deformities due to fat deposits, cellulite, stretch marks, leg veins, and the signs of aging on their hands and feet.

FAT PADS

Fat pads are localized areas of subcutaneous fat (under the skin) which affect the shapeliness of a person's body. Too much fat in a particular area can cause a contour deformity. Weight loss and exercise can significantly improve a less than desirable silhouette, however, these alternatives are not always enough. For this reason many individuals consider liposuction an acceptable solution. In fact it is the most popular cosmetic procedure in North America.

Liposuction

In the late 1970's, liposuction or suction lipolysis was developed so that localized fat could be surgically removed without leaving a significant scar. Since that time the procedure has been refined and developed to a degree of sophistication that provides consistently reliable results. The most recent innovation is referred to as the tumescent or wet technique. Older techniques will be referred to as dry techniques.

Most esthetic surgeons would agree that the tumescent technique is the procedure of choice because it is safer and provides a more satisfactory cosmetic result. The tumescent technique was developed by Dr. Jeffrey Klein, a dermatologist who wanted to reduce the risk of the procedure as well as improve the healing time and the cosmetic results of liposuction.

Who is a candidate for liposuction?

An ideal candidate for liposuction would be characterized as having:

- good elasticity of the skin so it will shrink adequately after the underlying fat has been removed.
- stable weight for 6 months prior to the surgery,
- good health,
- a regular exercise program,
- normal blood clotting,
- a tendency to heal well after injury, and
- realistic expectations.

Although the results of liposuction may contribute to an improvement in an individual's body image and self-esteem, it will not change or improve relationships or solve psychological problems.

What problems can liposuction correct?

Although exceptions exist, liposuction is designed for people who are close to their normal weight and have found that through diet and exercise they are unable to rid themselves of unwanted fat deposits. A typical example is the saddlebag or "riding breech" deformity on the upper outer thigh. This is often an inherited problem that persists despite vigorous exercise and dieting. The fat deposits collect in the hip, buttocks, and thigh areas creating a silhouette in the shape of a violin. This problem can be corrected with liposuction.

A more shapely and attractive leg can be created with liposuction by removing excess fat on the inner and outer thigh, the inside of the knee, and the upper portion of the calf and ankle. Liposuction is not limited to buttocks and limbs. As discussed in the previous chapter, fat may be removed from the abdomen of individuals who have good muscle tone and skin elasticity without the necessity of a tummy tuck. Similarly, liposuction of the neck, jowls, and cheeks gives a better profile without the need for more extensive surgery. The procedure can also be used for reduction of excess fat in the arms and in the lateral portion of the breasts.

Men appreciate the benefits of liposuction for reducing their love handles and pot bellies.

What is involved in a tumescent liposuction procedure?

First, a pre-operative consultation. During this initial visit the cosmetic surgeon will want to determine through discussion the desired outcome. A physical examination and body analysis will determine whether it is possible to achieve the results through liposuction. The physician will evaluate the fat deposits and underlying muscle

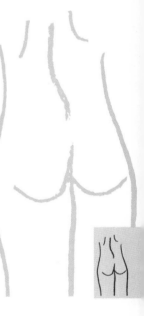

tone. They will also note any pre-existing scars, hernias, or asymmetry which may affect the outcome. To avoid disappointment this is the time for the patient and the physician to be totally honest. If a person's expectations are unrealistic it is better not to proceed.

Second, a pre-operative visit. During the pre-operative visit the patient is given all the necessary details related to the procedure including the pre-operative and post-operative instructions. A complete medical history and physical examination is performed. For the safety of the patient and the medical staff, pre-operative blood tests are done which include tests for HIV, hepatitis B, hepatitis C and blood stability.

Finally, on the day of the procedure:

■ Prior to beginning the procedure, the locations of the fat to be removed are mapped out on the skin with a permanent ink pen while the patient is standing so the effects of gravity can be noted. The effect is that of a topographical map on the skin and the ink takes a while to wash off after the procedure. A photograph is then taken.

■ At the discretion of the surgeon an anesthetist may be present to monitor the patient's vital signs but not to give an anesthetic. This is important when extensive procedures are

performed. A needle is inserted into the vein of one arm. It would be used as a vehicle to give fluids or medication if it were ever necessary. A blood pressure cuff is placed on the opposite arm. The analogy can be drawn that these precautions are like wearing a seat belt in the car. You wear the seat belt every day but you rarely if ever need it. When and if you do need it you are glad you had the foresight to use it routinely because you cannot predict when it might be required.

■ The incision sites are anesthetized and the incisions are made. Depending on the size of the fat deposit, several incisions may be required. Longer needles are then inserted through the incisions to introduce the medicated saline solution into the subcutaneous fat. The actual injection of the solution is almost painless. A slight prickling or aching sensation is experienced under the skin as the area becomes numb.

■ The bulk of the solution is made up of saline which is similar to the make up of the body's fluids. Four medications are added to the saline: lidocaine, epinephrine, bicarbonate and cortisone. Each contributes to a less traumatic form of surgery than the dry technique and ensures a faster, more comfortable healing time.

YOUNG AS YOU LOOK

Lidocaine is a local anesthetic which numbs the area to be treated such that general anesthetics, intravenous sedatives or narcotic analgesics are not necessary. The latter are generally used to some extent with the dry techniques. Post-operative discomfort is also minimized since the local anesthesia remains in the surgically treated areas for approximately 18 hours after surgery. Any further discomfort can be managed comfortably with an analgesic such as Tylenol.

Epinephrine, which temporarily shrinks capillaries, dramatically reduces both the bleeding during surgery and bruising after surgery. In fact, there is so little blood loss with the tumescent technique that often more blood loss is experienced from the pre-operative laboratory tests than during the actual liposuction surgery. Minimal bleeding shortens the post-operative recovery time. Most patients can return to work and begin exercising again within a day or two after surgery.

The tumescent solution is buffered with bicarbonate which brings the pH of the solution closer to that of the body. This helps to minimize the discomfort of the injections.

The mild cortisone controls inflammation which in turn results in less post-operative swelling and discomfort.

The tumescent technique also dictates the use of very small circular cannulas to suck out the fat as compared to large cannulas employed with the dry technique. The smaller cannulas allow the surgeon better control over the direction, depth and amount of fat removed during surgery. This reduces the risk of irregularities.

Because smaller cannulas are used, only small incisions are required. The incisions are so small that sutures are not necessary. The open incisions allow any excess tumescent solution to drain which helps to minimize bruising and soreness. An added benefit is that a smaller incision will heal faster.

■ A waiting period of 30 to 90 minutes takes place after the area has been well infiltrated with a large volume of tumescent solution. This allows the local anesthetic and blood vessel constrictor to take effect to ensure the area is completely numb and that bleeding will be minimal .

■ A suction cannula is inserted into the targeted layer of fat through the small incisions. The cannula is connected to a machine, via a tube, that provides a gentle suction force. As the cannula is pushed back and forth in several directions through the saline engorged fat, the fat is sucked into a reservoir bottle. This succession of forward and backward

Liposuction

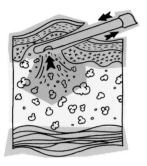

Fat is suctioned into cannula as it is moved back and forth.

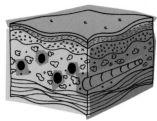

SKIN

FAT CELLS

MUSCLE

Liposuction tunnels are created in the fat.

motions of the cannula through the incision, creates numerous tunnels throughout the layer of fat. The surrounding fat collapses into the empty tunnels. The more tunnels created, the greater the fat reduction. The use of small cannulas with the tumescent technique offers better control over the direction and depth of the tunnels within the fat. It is important that the surgeon leaves a small layer of fat under the skin to avoid puckering and to maintain a soft, supple feel to the skin.

■ Once an adequate amount of fat has been removed, absorbent pads are placed over the tiny incisions and held in place by a pressure garment. The incisions are not sutured in order that the remaining solution can drain off into the pads. This helps minimize swelling, bruising and soreness.

■ Eighty percent of the tumescent solution is absorbed into the body and excreted in the urine and 20% is either sucked out with the fat or drained out through the tiny incision sites. The solution that drains from the incision is 98% saline solution and 2% blood. The blood gives the solution a red appearance. Drainage is greatest immediately after the procedure and gradually subsides over 2 to 4 days for larger areas and in 1 to 4 days for smaller areas such as under the chin. The absorbent pads are changed and worn until the drainage is complete then it is only necessary to wear the compression garment for a few more days. The compression garments may be worn longer, although the length of time they are worn does not affect the outcome of

CHAPTER

15

Y O U N G   A S   Y O U   L O O K

the procedure. Wearing it longer helps to resolve the swelling faster. Most patients wear their garments for 4 to 5 days. The compression headband used after liposuction to the neck and chin is worn for the first 24 hours then is only required at night for a 10 day period.

Will the surgery hurt?

The anesthetic in the solution numbs the area to be treated so little or no pain is felt during the procedure.

Due to the residual local anesthetic and the mild cortisone absorbed into the tissue, most patients do not experience any significant soreness for 6 to 18 hours after the procedure. An aching sensation similar to what might be felt after rigorous exercise may be experienced for 24 to 48 hours after the surgery. Maximum discomfort is generally experienced 5 days after surgery once the anti-inflammatory effect of the cortisone has worn off. Tylenol helps to control the inflammation thereby reducing this temporary discomfort.

Will there be a scar?

The wet or tumescent technique employs many 4 mm entry sites that heal rapidly and are not noticeable 6 months after the procedure. With the dry technique, one or several incisions 1 centimeter (1/2 inch) in length are made. After healing they leave a

fine pink scar which gradually fades into a white line within 6 months.

Could more than one area be treated at the same time?

Many areas may be treated at one time, although the limiting factor is the hemoglobin level. The more fat removed, the greater the drop in the red blood cell level. If a large amount of fat removal is anticipated, the procedure is often scheduled over a series of appointments in order to avoid the necessity of a blood transfusion.

When may normal activities be resumed?

Body movement and physical activity is encouraged after tumescent liposuction because it facilitates drainage of the residual solution.

Normal activities may be resumed within 48 hours of tumescent liposuction but activities should be restricted to 25% of that which would normally take place, then gradually built up to a full routine by the end of 1 or 2 weeks. This is compared to a recommended 2 weeks off work and 6 weeks off exercise when the dry technique is used.

Twenty four hours after tumescent liposuction a person may begin:

- driving a car,

- shopping,

- work, and

CHAPTER **15**

- exercise, including bicycling, golf, low impact aerobics, tennis, and walking. High impact sports should be delayed for a few weeks and integrated slowly into a daily routine of activities.

What are the possible complications of tumescent liposuction?

The complications associated with other cosmetic procedures, such as scarring, hematomas, and infections are rare with tumescent liposuction.

By magnifying the fatty compartment the tumescent technique permits more accurate removal of fat with greater assurance that the liposuction cannula will not approach the undersurface of the skin which could cause waves, dents, or dimples in the skin. If irregularities do occur they tend to subside within 6 months to a year. Cellulite is a contour deformity which may or may not lessen with liposuction. In fact, in some cases cellulite may become worse.

Asymmetry may also occur when more fat is removed from one side of the body than the other. This can easily be corrected by taking a bit more fat from the heavier side. If too much fat is removed, a droopy appearance in such areas as the buttocks might result.

Excessive bleeding and dehydration are risks associated with the dry liposuction technique.

The wet or tumescent technique significantly reduces these risks.

Other potential complications include:

- slight flushing of the face due to prostaglandin release from the fat, which usually occurs the day after the procedure,

- a slight temperature elevation shortly after the procedure,

- irregular or premature onset of menstruation which is presumed to be related to prostaglandin release,

- inflammation of the incision sites,

- collections of blood vessels on the skin,

- sensory nerve damage resulting in persistent discomfort or numbness,

- lymph channel interruption and varicose veins.

Mild speeding of the heart may result from the effects of the epinephrine in the tumescent solution. Some drugs such as thyroid supplements, appetite suppressants and the like may interact with the epinephrine to cause a faster heart rate.

Dr. William Hanke recently completed a survey that demonstrated the safety of the tumescent technique. Sixty-six dermatologic surgeons reported that there were no transfusions, hospitalizations or major complications in the 15,000 cases reviewed utilizing the tumescent technique. Nevertheless, side effects may occur even in the best of hands.

What are the limitations of liposuction?

Liposuction is not used for the treatment of generalized obesity. It is only effective in correcting unwanted fat in specific areas of the body. People who are generally over weight first need to commit to a lifestyle change which will encompass a proper diet and an exercise program. This for many is easier said than done and we recommend that expert assistance with this process is sought. Once a person reaches a reasonable weight and the remaining fat deposits are stable, liposuction may be considered for certain areas of the body.

Will liposuction get rid of stretch marks and cellulite?

Liposuction will not improve the appearance of stretch marks although treatments with topical tretinoin or laser resurfacing may be helpful.

In some cases liposuction may improve the appearance of cellulite. Creating a crisscross of tunnels through the fat with the very small cannulas used in tumescent liposuction causes mild inflammation of the fibrous pillars that hold the skin to the underlying muscular structure. As the inflammation subsides, the entire area contracts

down pulling the skin with it, much like a layer of Spandex . The more elasticity in the skin the greater the positive benefit of this contraction. Although liposuction is not used to treat cellulite, the effect of this tethering may help to improve the appearance of this condition if it is in an area where liposuction is done.

Should weight be lost before liposuction?

A person's body weight should remain stable for 6 months prior to surgery and should be maintained by weight management and exercise after the procedure is complete. Any excessive post-surgical weight gain will lay down a uniform layer of fat over the entire body. It will not accumulate in those areas treated as the number of fat cells in these areas have been reduced with liposuction and they do not grow back. Never the less, excessive weight gain is unattractive and to a certain extent will undo the results of the procedure. Weight loss after liposuction will, on the other hand, simply improve the esthetic results.

How does tumescent liposuction compare to the dry technique?

WET OR TUMESCENT TECHNIQUE

Swelling, bruising, inflammation and soreness are to be expected with the tumescent technique but

Hips Liposuction

BEFORE

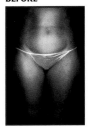

AFTER

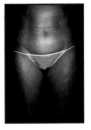

PHOTOS
COURTESY OF
DR. DON GROOT

CHAPTER 15

not to the extent that it occurs with the dry technique. The more fat that has been removed the longer the duration of post-operative swelling. Temporary subcutaneous lumpiness and firmness are also common during the healing process. This may persist to some degree for 2 to 6 months.

Bruising is usually minimal because there is less bleeding due to the presence of epinephrine in the tumescent solution. Factors which contribute to bruising include the extent of the area treated and an individual's unique tendency to bruise. If bruising occurs, it gradually subsides over a 10 to 15 day period.

It is common for patients to feel sore and be easily fatigued for a few days after tumescent liposuction. However, it is possible to return to all normal activities within 48 hours of the procedure.

In 90% of cases an improvement can actually be seen one week after tumescent liposuction. However, because of the slow resolution of post-surgical swelling, the ultimate results are realized in 12 to 24 weeks.

DRY TECHNIQUE

When the dry technique is used the suctioned area always bruises extensively. The bruising often extends well beyond the areas treated, and takes up to 3 weeks to disappear. For the first 3 to 6

weeks after the procedure, the area swells considerably. Massage and ultrasound therapy are often advised, and usually begin one week after the procedure for a period of 3 to 4 weeks. Massage seems to speed up the resolution of bruising and swelling and decreases the amount of fibrous tissue that might develop under the skin. Wearing supporting garments for 3 to 6 weeks following surgery also helps to diminish the bruising and swelling.

Due to the swelling, improvement will not be noticed immediately. For the first 3 weeks following liposuction with the dry technique, clothing is usually fairly snug, and disillusionment may set in because there is little change. Around the 6 week mark, clothing begins to fit more loosely. After approximately 3 months, swelling has subsided to the point that clothing one size smaller may be worn. Healing is usually complete 9 to 12 months after surgery, and a further reduction in clothing size is usually anticipated. This depends on the amount of fat removed.

Fatigue may set in during the first few weeks following surgery. This may be due to a drop in hemoglobin as a result of bruising and iron supplements may be recommended. The amount of fat removed at the time of surgery is controlled to ensure that the red blood cell count does not drop to dangerously low levels which

YOUNG AS YOU LOOK

would necessitate a blood transfusion.

Two weeks off work is recommended and no exercise should be done for 6 weeks.

What is ultrasonic liposuction?

Ultrasonic liposuction is a relatively new technique where sound waves are passed along the cannula causing emulsification of the fat prior to aspiration. This allows the surgeon to get closer to the skin surface while reducing the risk of troughing and wrinkling. Many surgeons feel the ultrasonic technique provides an added dimension of safety in high volume fat removal, particularly when combined with the tumescent technique. It also provides an added advantage over other techniques in areas of the body that are fibrous such as the ankles, upper back and breasts in men (gynaecomastia) and areas of the body that are poorly supported by underlying muscle such as the inner thighs.

One of the disadvantages of this technique in the past was the overheating of the cannula which in some cases burned the skin. The latest equipment has a device which wraps around the cannula circulating water to keep it cool. It also has a pressure monitoring system to control for excess vibration and potential heat build up which could damage the skin.

The technique is performed under local or general anesthetic at the discretion of the surgeon and patient. The ultrasonic instrumentation is tenfold the cost of traditional liposuction equipment and this as well as the lengthy nature of the procedure escalates the costs of the surgery.

What are the alternatives to liposuction?

Dieting to obtain an ideal weight, in combination with a regular exercise program, is the cornerstone to maintaining a healthy and attractive physical form. For many individuals, however, the ideal is not possible because of persistent deposits of fat that detract from their physical appearance. For these victims of fat liposuction is a potential solution.

What is microlipid transfer?

Microlipid transfer is the process by which fat is injected into areas of fat deficiency. This fat is harvested from the products of liposuction, cleansed, and then reinjected. The short term results are quite satisfactory, but in the long-term, relocated fat is almost always progressively metabolized.

Who performs liposuction and how much does it cost?

Dermatologists and plastic surgeons trained in liposuction techniques perform these procedures. In some centers, specialists other than plastic surgeons or dermatologists will also perform liposuction. It is

CHAPTER 15

up to the individual to ensure that the surgeon is qualified, board certified, well trained, and experienced in any procedure being considered.

For the first anatomic area the cost ranges from $2,000 to $6,000. For each subsequent area the cost is usually $2,000 to $5,000. An anatomic area represents both the right and left side of the body: for example the right and left hip or the right and left thigh.

CELLULITE

Most women who have cellulite would concur that it is almost indestructible. Maintaining a low body weight and lower fat stores helps but is no guarantee that this problem will not creep into your life with advancing age.

Heredity and hormonal changes play a role in the creation of this localized change to the smooth skin surface of the thighs and buttocks. The connections between the coating of the muscle and the skin stretch in some areas and contract in others creating a fibrous mesh. The fatty layer between the skin and the muscle thickens and pushes out of the holes in the mesh creating the uneven cobblestone appearance of cellulite.

Heat generating massaging creams, superficial suction devices, and electronic muscle stimulators are some of the techniques for which claims have been made that

they work to reduce cellulite. It is doubtful, however, whether these techniques provide permanent results. They irritate and inflame the superficial tissue resulting in an accumulation of fluid (or edema). This layer of fluid behaves like a water cushion in the skin's second layer (over the fatty third layer). This effectively masks the cellulite, temporarily disguising but not solving the problem. The effect is similar to that of agents used to cause irritation, fluid shifts, and swelling of the skin to temporarily puff up and iron out wrinkles.

Unfortunately, there is no long term solution to cellulite. However there is some hope. A preparation known as aminophylline cream applied to the affected area twice a day reduces cellulite in some people. At this time aminophylline cream is only available through a prescription. It is not an over the counter preparation so do not go searching for it on the shelves of the local pharmacy. The regular use of this cream in combination with the following suggestions should help to improve the look of the thighs and buttocks of women afflicted with cellulite:

■ Maintaining lower fat stores with a well balanced low fat diet.

■ Avoiding anything that encourages deep fluid retention, such as too much salt in the diet and too many diet drinks. In this case, the hormonal balance should also be evaluated.

YOUNG AS YOU LOOK

- Tone the muscles with daily buttocks, hip, and thigh exercises so that the fat cushion is sitting on a firm base. Exercises such as vigorous walking, swimming, and cycling are particularly helpful.

- Vigorously massage the areas of cellulite for 10 minutes each day to break down the fibrous mesh and the larger fat globules. Applying a hot water bottle or heating pad to the area prior to vigorously manipulating the area with aggressive judo chops will help, but care must be taken not to overheat and burn the skin. Follow the massage with an ice pack.

If all else fails and you are desperate a combination of surgical liposuction to remove fat from the bulges and fat transfer to place fat in the dimples may even out irregularities and permanently remove some of the fat stores.

STRETCH MARKS

To minimize the possibility of stretch marks, care should be taken to avoid unnecessary and prolonged use of potent cortisone skin preparations which weaken the skin and predispose it to stretch marks. Excessive weight fluctuations and use of muscle building steroids during physical training should also be avoided.

Stretch marks are unsightly and a cosmetic solution is commonly sought. To date, this condition has been difficult to treat. Vitamin E oil, aloe vera, and similar agents do not prevent or reverse this problem, and allergic reactions to these agents are common. Many techniques currently being used to reduce or eliminate stretch marks are not yet refined and require further exploration and research.

What is the best available treatment for stretch marks?

The use of tretinoin has proven to be the most effective treatment to date. Tretinoin in the form of Retisol-A, Retin-A, Stieva-A, Rejuva-A, Renova or Vitamin A Acid applied to stretch marks in high doses causes a realignment of the collagen in the skin.

To be effective, tretinoin must be applied in a high dosage, no less than 0.1% per day, for a period of twelve weeks. The area becomes very irritated, dry and itchy. This reaction is important to the success of the treatment and must not be interfered with by using moisturizing creams or mild cortisone creams to improve the discomfort.

Researchers have found that 4 out of 20 people find they cannot tolerate the irritation. Of the remaining numbers; 25% demonstrate a complete reversal of their stretch marks, 70% experience some improvement and 5% show no improvement at all. Stretch marks that have developed recently are more receptive to treatment with tretinoin than stretch marks which have been around for awhile. (Tretinoin has been discussed in detail in Chapter 6).

Are there other alternatives for the treatment of stretch marks?

Yes, there are other options, but they are not as effective as the application of tretinoin. The next best alternative is to resurface the stretch marks with the carbon dioxide laser. As with tretinoin, this causes a reorganization of the collagen architecture in the skin. Up to 75% improvement has been noted with this technique, but complete reversal of the stretch marks has not been achieved. Also, the treated area may remain red or pink for as long as 1 or 2 years. Care must be taken, as overly aggressive laser treatments may result in scarring and irregular pigmentation.

In some cases the vascular removal lasers may help to improve the look of stretch marks. Lasers and how they work have been discussed in Chapter 7.

Another option is the use of injectable collagen. Zyplast collagen can be injected and moulded into the depressed and thinned areas of the stretch marks. The results are variable and not permanent, and the amount of collagen that would be required to fill large areas of stretch marks would be very costly.

These factors do not make this an attractive alternative for most individuals. (For detailed information about injectable collagen refer to Chapter 6).

Linear surgical excision may help in select instances where a fine white scar would be preferable to unsightly stretch marks.

Opaque cosmetics, such as Covermark and Dermablend, may be used to camouflage visible stretch marks if they are particularly troublesome.

LEG VEINS

Depending on what is worn, the legs are quite visible, and leg veins often stand out. Women suffer more from this condition than men. Fortunately, much can be done to eliminate this problem. Spider veins are small superficial veins which will not disappear by themselves; they must be treated.

What can be done to prevent leg veins?

The following preventative measures may be taken to control conditions such as spider and varicose veins:

■ Avoid standing in one spot for long periods. Contraction of the calf muscle through movement acts like a pump to aid the blood in returning back to the heart. Swelling and dilation of leg veins are less likely to produce varicose veins if the muscle contractions are frequent.

■ If the blood vessels are large, support hose should be worn to help prevent dilation of these vessels. Be careful to avoid the tourniquet effect that often occurs when knee-high or thigh-length stockings are worn.

■ Lose weight. A large stomach will press on the larger veins in the pelvis creating unnecessary back pressure and stress on the veins of the legs.

■ Do not cross the legs as this inhibits the flow of blood from the legs to the heart.

■ Elevate the feet higher than the ankles when convenient. At night, put the end of the bed on wooden blocks. This places the body at an angle which encourages the blood in the leg veins to return to the heart.

■ Avoid high impact aerobics which can dilate veins. Other forms of aerobic exercise, such as cycling, rowing, swimming, and vigorous walking can help in two ways. First, it improves muscle tone and thereby the muscle pump. Second, the massaging effect of this type of exercise encourages the blood and tissue fluid of the legs into circulation away from the legs towards the heart.

What can be done to get rid of spider veins?

For very fine blushes of blood vessels on the legs the pulsed dye laser can be used, however for larger more defined vessels sclerotherapy is the treatment of choice. Recently, the variable pulse width (VPW) laser and other nonlaser light sources have been used to eradicate smaller leg veins. Success varies with laser removal of leg veins and cannot be guaranteed. The pulse dye laser and the VPW lasers are discussed in detail in Chapter 7.

For years, solutions have been injected into large and small veins of the legs causing them to shrink and become less obvious. This procedure is known as sclero-therapy. The irritating solution causes the lining of the vein to become inflamed and the walls to adhere to each other. The vein shrinks and disappears from sight.

A number of irritating solutions (or sclerosants), in various concentrations, are used. They include morrhate sodium (Scleromate), concentrated salt solutions (hypertonic saline), concentrated sugar solutions (dextrose), a blend of salt, sugar, and alcohol (Dextroject, Sclerodex), polidocanol solution (Aethoxy-sklerol, Sclerovein), and Sotradechol solution.

Sclerotherapy is a helpful procedure for women and men

CHAPTER 15

with unsightly and often aching lower limbs. It is usually tolerated well and serious side effects are rare. Sclerotherapy can be used in other areas where spider veins may occur, including the chest, the nose, and the back of the hands. Facial injections, however, have a greater associated risk because of the vascular connections to the eyes and brain. Vascular lasers such as the flashlamp pulsed dye and the variable pulse width lasers are much more effective and safer in treating veins on the face and chest.

True varicose veins, particularly if they are large, may require surgical stripping and ligation procedures.

What is involved in sclerotherapy?

- Usually sclerotherapy requires that the patient lies on her back or abdomen but various body positions may be necessary so the physician can accurately inject the sclerosant into the spider veins.

- The area to be treated is cleansed and a small needle is introduced into the "trunk" of the venous "tree" from which the small branches of vessels emerge; then the sclerosant is injected into the vessel. As soon as the sclerosant enters the vein, it turns white. This is an important clue to the physician

that the sclerosant has entered the vein. The needle is then removed and pressure applied to the injection site.

- A potent cortisone cream may be applied immediately after the injection to minimize redness and swelling. Pressure dressings are used if the vessels are medium to large in diameter.

- As many as 50 sites are injected depending on the size of each spider vein grouping.

What happens after sclerotherapy?

Immediately after the injections the areas treated are red, bruised, and swollen; this gradually subsides over a 3 week period. In some cases iron stains from the blood may leave a residual brown color, which may take several weeks or months to disappear.

The vein is visible for several days after the injection, then gradually fades away completely.

Rest, with the legs elevated, is advised for 2 to 3 days after the procedure, and jarring exercises and long periods of standing should be avoided for 1 week. In reality many people do not have the time or luxury to take advantage of this advice, yet usually do well regardless. It is important to protect the legs from sun exposure after the injections; otherwise discoloration is more likely to occur. Opaque cosmetic coverage will camouflage any redness, bruising, and possible hyper-pigmentation. Bleaching creams such as Reversa HQ and NeoStrata HQ help to control residual pigmentation, and the earlier they are used, the better.

How successful is sclerotherapy?

Over 90% of patients who undergo sclerotherapy are satisfied. The cure and healing of the vessels depends on the following factors: the size of the injected vessels, the type and concentration of the sclerosant, the skill of the operator, the post-procedural care, and the nature of the vessels. Although new spider veins may appear, the injected veins usually do not return.

Does sclerotherapy hurt?

Most patients find it only mildly uncomfortable, although for some the needle pricks, itching, and cramping are quite uncomfortable, particularly if large amounts of concentrated salt solutions are used. If the injection misses the vein and the sclerosant is injected into the skin beside a vessel, a burning sensation is felt. The legs often ache for the first few days after a series of injections.

What complications can sclerotherapy cause?

The complications which may occur are best described as nuisance complications because they are not serious and are dealt with easily. They include:

■ Infection at the injection site, which can be treated with topical antibiotics such as Fucidin ointment.

■ Distal angioplasias are very tiny mats or flushes of vessels near the injection site that were not there at the time of the injection.

Fortunately, they usually resolve with time. The potential for these occurring increases if the patient is taking estrogen, if the sclerosant has been injected under pressure, if large amounts of the sclerosant was required, or if the compression dressings were put on too tightly.

■ If the vessels do not disappear, they are reinjected with a larger amount or a higher concentration of the same or a different sclerosant. In some cases the VPW laser is used.

■ As with any drug, a local or a generalized allergic reaction may occur, such as a skin rash or breathing difficulty.

■ Phlebitis and fibrotic nodules (vein inflammation and scarring bumps) are common even in small blood vessels, and are

CHAPTER 15

really part of the expected response which is resolved over time. Fortunately, they are usually mild, superficial, and uncomplicated. In rare instances, when large veins are sclerosed, a thrombosis may occur. This is more serious since blood clots might travel to the lungs and cut off the vital supply of oxygen to the body. This is virtually unheard of when small vessels are treated.

■ Asthma attacks may occur when Aethoxysklerol is used. This agent should not be injected into the veins of patients with severe bronchial asthma.

Who should not have sclerotherapy?

Contraindications include a history of deep vein thrombophlebitis. Pregnant women, patients on prolonged bed rest, people taking anticoagulants, or those who are known to have allergies to any of the sclerosant agents need to be carefully screened.

How much does sclerotherapy cost and who performs it?

Sclerotherapy costs between $100 and $200 per session, depending on the number of vessels that need to be injected. Usually 2 to 6 sessions are required, but more extensive problems may require up to 15 sessions. Dermatologists and registered nurses under the guidance of a dermatologist

commonly treat small spider veins, whereas general surgeons treat the larger veins.

AGING HANDS AND FEET

"You can tell a woman's age by her hands" is a common saying. Until recently this was true, but no longer. The single biggest factor which contributes to a hand looking aged is age spots.

Age Spots

Age spots, known medically as lentigos and seborrhoeic keratoses, are brown patches which commonly appear on the back of the hands, the face, and the back. Heredity and sun exposure are largely responsible for this excess melanin production in the skin. Several treatment options are available to rid the body of age spots.

Cryotherapy: Until recently the treatment of choice for age spots was cryotherapy. With this technique liquid nitrogen is sprayed very gently on the spots to induce a localized frostbite. After two or three weeks the treated age spot peels off as the underlying skin pushes to the surface, leaving a residual area of pinkness that might last for only a week but could linger on for months. Scarring may occur.

Laser therapy: With the advent of the pigment removal lasers

YOUNG AS YOU LOOK

(Q-switched ruby, Alexandrite, and Nd:Yag), cryotherapy is no longer the treatment of choice, because the laser has a lower risk of scarring, is less painful and the recovery time is shorter. Due to the cost of laser treatments and because not all physicians have access to a laser nor are they trained in laser surgery, many individuals still choose cryotherapy to treat their age spots. The pigment removal lasers have also superseded the use of surgical removal or vaporization with the carbon dioxide laser for larger growths provided they are not too thick. If the lesion is suspected to be cancerous then a biopsy is always taken prior to proceeding with laser surgery so it can be analyzed by a pathologist. If it is malignant then surgical removal is used to ensure that the cancer has been completely removed. The carbon dioxide laser in its cutting mode may be used to do the surgical excision.

The pigment removal lasers act in a similar fashion to a guided missile. The light from the laser has a selective affinity for brown dis-coloration in the skin. It passes harmlessly through the top layer of skin and when it hits the brown pigment cells energy is released causing the melanosomes in the cell to break into minuscule particles which are removed by the body's immune system.

Each pulse of laser light feels like the snap of an elastic band on the skin. The age spot turns grey initially, then within minutes forms a superficial brown crust. Within 2 weeks the crust will be sloughed and the skin underneath will be pink. This gradually fades to the color of the surrounding skin over the course of 2 to 3 weeks. It takes less time for age spots to turn over on the face than on the back of the hands. The crusts must not be picked or rubbed off otherwise a scar will result.

Bleaching Creams:
Prescription bleaching creams containing kojic acid or hydro-quinone cause age spots and irregular pigmentation to fade so that they blend with the color of the surrounding skin. Reversa HQ and NeoStrata HQ are examples of over-the-counter gels containing glycolic acid and bleaching agents which are effective in lightening age spots and other irregular pigmentation in the skin. It is important to protect yourself against the sun with a broad spectrum sunscreen such as Ombrelle 15, otherwise you will defeat the purpose of the bleaching creams.

Medicated Creams:
Tretinoin in preparations such as Retin-A, Stieva-A, Rejuva-A, Retisol-A, Renova and Vitamin A Acid, when applied to the back of the hands daily over a period of months gradually causes age spots

to disappear, evens out irregular pigmentation, and reduces fine wrinkles giving the hands a more youthful appearance.

Chemical Peels:

Acid containing solutions are also effective in removing age spots. They cause irritation and the spots peel away from the skin. The new underlying skin is pink and fades to a normal hue after a few months.

Camouflage Makeup:

Opaque makeup can be used daily to camouflage age spots. Given the excellent medical options for removing or lightening these dis-colorations of the skin, makeup becomes a less desirable alternative.

Older Looking Hands

What about the bony look that older hands tend to have?

The depressions which appear between the ligaments on the backs of the hands with age are due to fat redistribution and a loss of elasticity in the skin. If this is truly troublesome to some individuals they can be filled with a soft tissue implant such as collagen or fat. The pros and cons of soft tissue implants have been discussed in Chapter 6. Large veins on the back of the hands cannot be avoided, however small spider-like veins can be erased with sclerotherapy or with a vascular removal laser if the veins are blush-like in appearance.

Sclerotherapy involves the injection of a salt and sugar solution (sclerosants) into the veins which causes the wall of the vein to scar off preventing blood from flowing through it. Details of this treatment have been discussed in this chapter under leg veins.

The vascular removal lasers, as another treatment option, send a light into the skin which acts like a missile targeting red discolorations in the skin. In this fashion it causes the blood cells to break up so they can be carried away by macrophage cells and to seal the vessels.

Nails

Nail enhancing techniques (out-lined in the *Chapter 2: The Hair and Nails*) are useful for daily care of the nails. Rough, cracked, and irregular nails improve if soaked in warm water for 10 minutes twice daily, and if water absorbing creams are applied to the moist nails. These chemically enhanced moisturizers (such as Lachydrin, Lacticare, Uremol, Calmurid) contain urea and/or lactic acid.

A glass slide used for micro-scopic work, and available from a dermatologist, may be used to smooth and sculpt the nails by rubbing it back and forth across the surface of the nails causing an erosion of the rough, irregular, or prominent areas.

YOUNG AS YOU LOOK

Calcium and gelatin supplements do not strengthen nails despite earlier unsupported claims to the contrary.

Nails often reflect internal medical problems such as heart, liver, and/or kidney disease, as well as subtle changes in early iron and thyroid deficiencies, and internal infection. Therefore, unusual problems with nails should be investigated by a physician.

Regular manicures with a qualified esthetician help to keep the hands looking young and attractive.

Palms and Soles

Dry, fissured and cracked heels and palms improve when soaked in warm water, patted dry, and covered with a chemically enhanced moisturizer such a

Uremol 10 or Norwegian Hand Formula lotion while the hands and feet are still moist. The urea and other agents in these moisturizers act like a sponge to hold the moisture in the skin.

Open fissures may be irritated by creams which contain urea or lactic acid. To prevent this discomfort, vaseline may be applied to cuts after soaking and before applying these moisturizers. To speed up softening of the skin, wrap the soaked and creamed hands or feet in plastic sandwich wrap such as Saran Wrap and wear socks or gloves over them during the night. After removing the plastic wraps or after soaking, use a pumice stone on calloused skin.

Pedicures by a qualified esthetician on a regular basis help to keep the feet smooth and comfortable, as well as attractive.

CHAPTER 15

Your
Personal
Style

The *Final Touch*

FINE TUNING YOUR SELF-IMAGE

What do you feel when you catch a reflection of your body in a window or a mirror?

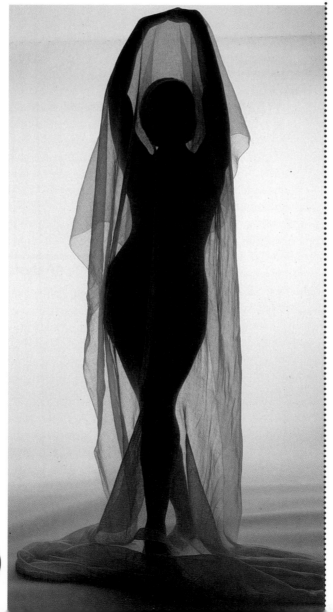

Turn your attention to the way you dress. Certain lines, colors, and fabric weights will either accentuate a well cared for physique or detract from the effort that has been put into creating a terrific look.

*C*onsciously boost that self-image 25 to 50% by thinking and dressing up to a positive self-image.

Our agenda for the final touch:

■ *body analysis*
■ *fabric line, weight, and color*
■ *personalized wardrobe*
■ *accessories*

BEING FASHIONABLE

Fashionable, definition: being observant of and conforming to the present fashion or style.

To be fashionable, according to this definition, is to adopt the yearly and seasonal trends. For most women and men this is unrealistic. The logical approach to creating a fashionable image is to choose the fashion that best suits you. Buying trendy items should be at the bottom of your priority list, and if the latest trend is not suitable for your body type, do not buy it.

Hem lines have been giving women mixed messages for years. The 1960's introduced the mini, and 30 years later it was here again. How to deal with it? Very simply, if a present trend does not look or feel good, do not wear it. Similar principles apply to men regarding the lines and "cut" of suit jackets.

No one can talk you into buying "the very latest" unless you let them. Take into consideration your size, shape, and personality when deciding on the latest styles. It is also appropriate to dress your age. This does not mean stifling your sense of fashion and becoming sombre and dull, but rather, moving into a more classic mode of dressing and leaving the trendier items for the very young.

Think of yourself as a total package. Do not concentrate on one area and neglect the others. Your head-to-toe image includes a healthy lifestyle, good skin care, an attractive hair style, effective make-up, a positive personality, and clothing that is right for you. A little knowledge is no danger, the basics count for a lot.

Body Analysis

By analyzing your body, you can see which are your attractive and unattractive features. Body analysis applies to both women and men. Start with a full-length mirror and a few basic questions. A woman might ask the following:

■ Am I short (under 5'3"), average (5'4" to 5'6"), or tall (5'7" and above)?

■ Am I thin, average, or overweight? Being too thin is almost as unattractive as being too heavy. Will losing weight create a more balanced

CHAPTER 16

264   *YOUNG AS YOU LOOK*

proportion (that is, the top half as wide as or slightly wider than the bottom half)?

- What about my posture? Is it as good as it should be? Are my shoulders erect without being stiff? Is my tummy flat or protruding? Is my bottom flat, large, or sway-back?

- Are my shoulders square, sloping, too narrow, or too wide?

- Is my bust line too small, average, or too heavy for the rest of my body?

- Do I have a waistline? Does my waistline divide me into equal proportions or am I short or long waisted?

- Are my legs long, average, or short? Do my legs have definition? Are my ankles slim or thick?

- Are my arms average, top-heavy, or too thin?

- Finally, am I tall enough for my present width? Are my hips wider than my shoulders?

Analyze your figure front and back. If you are not sure, ask a friend to assist, but start at the top and work all the way down.

Be realistic! Wishing and hoping is not the answer. Work with what you have got and if it is less than perfect, learn to work around it.

Being familiar and comfortable with your own body shape is the key to presenting a fashionable image.

Fabric Line, Weight, and Color

At some point in your life you are affected by fashion and, therefore, require some basic knowledge of clothing and how draping affects your appearance. Through trial and error, you will eventually develop your own sense of style. It should be dictated by who you are, who you want to be, and who you want others to think you are.

Clothing is, very simply, a combination of line, color, and fabric weight, and everyone has to discover the best combination for his or her body type.

Clothing Line

The line of your clothing is important because subconsciously the eye follows these lines. Line is also what dermatologists and plastic surgeons consider in cosmetic surgical alterations of the physique. Designers use three lines (or combinations thereof) when designing the cut of a garment: vertical, diagonal, and horizontal. Not only does the line refer to fabric pattern but also to the overall cut and style.

The diagonal line is usually flattering for all figure types. It creates the illusion of slimness and can camouflage such figure faults

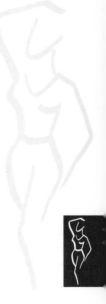

as heavy hips or shoulders and hips that appear, otherwise, too lean. Diagonal styling would de-emphasize a large bust line or prominent tummy. Examples of diagonal detailing are: lapel angle and width; pocket detailing on jackets, skirts, and trousers; criss-cross blouse or shirt front, and upper dress detailing; and the flattering effect created with the gentle drape of a large scarf or shawl over the shoulders.

Be wary of horizontal lines unless you are tall and slim. The petite and fine featured can use this line to broaden a small frame. Ruffles, flounces, wide collars, and added shoulder detailing will camouflage a small bust line or widen narrow shoulders. The horizontal line, however, is usually worn incorrectly. Anyone wanting to camouflage broad shoulders, heavy bust line, heavy arms, thick waistline, broad hips or derriere, or short heavy legs and ankles must always avoid horizontal detailing.

Watch Out For:

- short, puffy sleeves and short sleeves with cuffs;

- bodice detailing, ruffles, flounces, stripes;

- too much shoulder padding;

- patch pockets on jackets, trousers, and skirts;

- slacks with cuffs;

- pleated skirts, gathered waistlines;

- double-breasted jackets, blazers, and coats;

- patterns, plaids, or color schemes running horizontally;

- ankle straps on shoes;

- strong, contrasting colors dividing the body in half.

People want to create the illusion of height, slimness, and balanced proportion. In order to do this, you must dress in lines that fool the eye or enhance what you've got.

The vertical cut, color scheme, or pattern is by far the most complimentary. The eye moves up and down, not resting anywhere too long.

Vertical detailing:

- dressing in one color tone, including stockings, shoes, and handbag;

- V-necks and turtlenecks (not for the short neck, though!);

- vertical striping and stitching design;

- vertical tucking or pleating (if it is scaled down);

- low-buttoned, single-breasted suit jacket;

- front-pleated slacks with accentuated vertical folds or creases.

CHAPTER 16

The vertical line combined with the diagonal will do wonders for many figure faults, and is the easiest way to achieve a proportioned body image. This is probably one reason why uniforms and both low-buttoned single or even double-breasted suits are often so flattering on men.

The easiest way to increase shoulder width to balance hip width is by adding shoulder pads, a wonderful trick for both women and men if used subtly. Keep two or three sets handy, adding them under sweaters, blouses, T-shirts, dresses, or jackets so that shoulders are about one inch wider than the hip outline in women and two inches wider in men. The small-busted woman can augment her bust size with a slightly padded bra, horizontal detailing, or bold color scheme across the bust line. In this fashion, she effectively adds bulk to her upper body. The woman who wishes to camouflage a heavy hip and waist should avoid line detail as much as possible in that area. Do not use belts unless they are very narrow. An excellent dress line would be the chemise, an easy fit, falling straight from the shoulder.

In men, the "Continental suit" style de-emphasizes the waist. Avoid pockets unless they are vertically placed. Jumpsuits are also a style option to understate the male waistline.

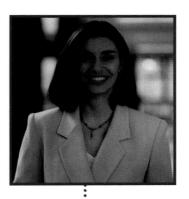

For the woman undergoing breast augmentation or reduction, tummy tuck, liposuction, or weight reduction, use of the three visual lines will affect the perception of her new body shape. She should delete the horizontal and incorporate the diagonal and vertical until her body shape is such that the horizontal is attractive and figure flattering for her. She should also pay particular attention to overall proportion.

The principles of line are applicable to men's clothing as well. Men should pay particular attention to jacket detailing: lapel placement and width, pleated versus plain trousers, cuffs versus no cuffs on slacks. Back vents in jackets should never pull open. Heavy-set men should avoid vents in jackets altogether or opt for side venting. Shoulder padding is very important in jackets to give a clean, tapered line. The man with a heavy midsection should consider wearing suspenders but care should be taken that the suspenders do not frame the tummy and draw attention to it. Suspenders may create a vertically clean line and prevent trousers from bagging above the shoes.

Men's clothing is generally freer of detail than women's, thereby

CHAPTER 16

simplifying the choice. Avoid plaids, large prints, and horizontal striping if your body frame or shape is heavy-set. Not unlike women, men want their overall appearance to be complimentary and flattering to their body size. Good features should be enhanced and weak ones minimized.

Fabric Weight

To create the illusion that you are tall, in proportion, and slim, you must consider fabric weight in your clothing purchases. Fabric can add weight. Heavy textures, such as mohair, heavy wools, wool plaids, boucles, knits, and large prints are bulky and can make you look big. Very fine fabrics, such as silk, silk jersey, chiffon, and silk crepe, tend to cling and outline your silhouette. Fabrics of medium weight, such as gabardines, polyester blends, cotton, fine wool, knits, wool crepe, linen, and silk blends, should be selected for most figure types.

Fabric Color

Color is able to contribute to a cohesive, workable wardrobe. The key to successful dressing is having clothing that is interchangeable, creating a variety of looks to meet most dress requirements. The only way to achieve this is to have a core foundation built around one or two color schemes, preferably in earth tones, cream, beige, taupe,

brown, black, grey, navy, olive, and khaki.

For women these basic colors (or neutrals) should form a foundation consisting of a coat, a jacket or blazer, one or two skirts, one or two pants, a dress, a tailored blouse, a dressier blouse, and one or two sweaters, depending on your lifestyle and daily needs. Seven to eleven interchangeable pieces are adequate in your favorite color scheme, but keep in mind that these pieces should be versatile and not too memorable so they may be worn more often. Men's wardrobes should reflect similar concepts. Color choice is of utmost importance; it should not be too strong, since the eye focuses on the most outstanding feature of an outfit. Use splashes of brighter color in accessories (ties, hankies, scarves, belts, jewelry, or sweaters) but only if your figure type will accommodate it.

Tone-on-tone dressing is always wise for all figure types, since it is the easiest and best way to create an uninterrupted vertical line. Repeated colors in your wardrobe must be good ones; they must be flattering to your skin type, hair color, and personality. Bright colors attract attention and might make you look bigger. Here are some examples of the effect color has on appearance:

■ Black can be an excellent foundation color but must be

YOUNG AS YOU LOOK

counterbalanced with proper makeup and hair color.

■ Greys and yellows can drain certain skin coloring; experiment with the shade and intensity of these colors.

■ Brown by itself can be boring but paired with cream or taupe it may look stunning.

■ Red is an exciting color but not for a person with a ruddy complexion. Red is often best used as an accent in gloves, belts, scarves, handbags, and shoes.

■ Pastels are soft colors and look very attractive on many figure and skin types.

Use color in various strengths and intensities to enhance figure type or to subdue undesirable body traits. Colors should complement skin type and personality. Well chosen color schemes give you a pleasing head-to-toe image.

A Personalized Wardrobe

Clothing is one of the strongest ways in which you can express yourself as an individual. Your personality affects your choices. Develop your own sense of style. Be comfortable.

Most men and women are a combination of two, and even three, personality types. When the occasion requires a certain look, they can dress appropriately and with credibility. Some body types are better suited to certain styles than others, so face the reality revealed by your mirror. Dress to enhance who you are and what you have.

Get into the habit of buying at least one fashion magazine a month. A good one for men is Gentlemen's Quarterly, and for women, Vogue. Study the looks, the clothes, and the way they are worn. Learn to read fashion pictures and check the details, however small they may seem.

Reading a fashion photo:

■ On a single- or double-breasted suit: how low is the button? How wide is the lapel?

■ Are the sleeves of a blouse, T-shirt, or jacket pushed up or rolled back?

■ Is the collar turned up or down?

■ Is the jacket belted, loose, buttoned or unbuttoned?

■ What kind of tops are tucked into skirts and slacks? Which are left loose? Which are belted?

■ How is the scarf tied?

■ Is the tie knotted in a tight single or double knot?

■ Study accessories (bangles, earrings, cuff links, pearls, chains, brooches, belts, watches, hair accessories, shoes, and tie tacks). Note how they are being worn.

CHAPTER 16

Accessories

Accessories include everything except the garment. They supply the final touch and need to be given careful consideration. Accessories should never dominate your outfit but should instead provide a point of interest. Some people avoid accessories altogether while others never know when to stop. Take a look in a full-length mirror and ask yourself: do I need more, less, or simply some re-adjusting of accessory wear?

Do these accessories enhance my overall appearance or are they drawing attention to a part of me that should be ignored?

The wonderful thing about accessories is that they can instantly update last year's favorite outfits and garments. People with a limited budget can use accessories to their advantage. Think of creating a vertical line with accessories and follow the well-known rule: when in doubt, leave it out.

Your
Personal
Program

IT
IS
YOUR
TURN

*Yes, it is
your turn.
You deserve
it, want it
and need it.
But how do
you carry
your
personal
program to
completion?*

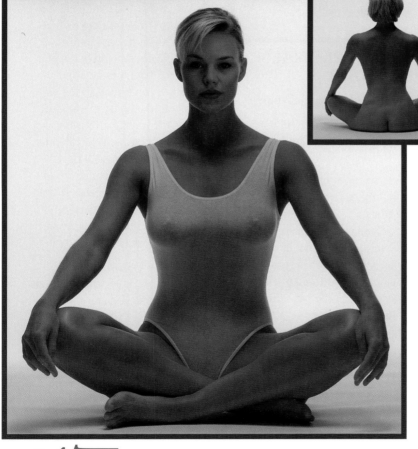

CHAPTER 17

*O*ur agenda for achieving your goals includes:

▪ *enjoying a healthy self-image*

▪ *the mind-body connection*

▪ *making a change*
  - *analyzing your needs*
  - *outlining your priorities*
  - *initiating a plan of action*
  - *eight steps to a healthy, attractive you!*

YOUR PERSONAL PROGRAM

Enjoying a Healthy Self-image

A healthy self-image contributes to the way we look and if we look good, we feel good about ourselves.

Most people at one time or another in their lives suffer from poor self-esteem, some more than others. Maintaining a strong, healthy self-esteem is not always easy in a society that has high expectations for performance and attractiveness. Yet life has so much more to offer to those who have a healthy sense of self.

Large sections of bookstores are dedicated to self-help books, many of which deal with how to bolster your self-esteem. It is not within the scope of this book to deal with the subject matter in-depth. From our own experience we can share a few helpful hints. If these do not provide you with the guidance you need then we suggest that you seek help from other sources, be it other books or a visit to a psychologist. Do not get stuck in a quagmire. As the song goes, "There is such a lot of living to do."

Enjoy who you are. Like your finger prints, you are unique. No one else is exactly like you. The way you laugh and smile, the way you view the world, the way you think, are uniquely yours.

Believe that your uniqueness is important. If all of us looked the same, thought the same and dressed the same, the world would be a boring place indeed. Your uniqueness contributes to the vast and beautiful tapestry of our world, and as such you are a valuable member of humanity. Not all of us will be famous or make a huge lasting mark on the world, but to those who come in contact with us, we will make an impression on their lives. And their uniqueness will make an impression on our lives.

Accept your uniqueness. Accept who you are, as you are, right now while preparing and planning for change and growth in the future. Growth and change are an inevitable part of living. At 20 you are a drastically different person from when you were 12, and you will be different at 40 and at 60. Your view of the world will grow and change with your life experiences and the knowledge you acquire along the way.

Enhance your uniqueness. Cultivate an interesting personality. Experience life. Seek out adventure or take on a new challenge.

Do not be afraid of change. At this moment in time you may not be happy with some aspect of your self-image. You may think that you are too heavy or out of shape. Maybe you believe that you are too quiet, or too loud. Maybe you are unhappy with some of your life choices. Accept where you are now, knowing that nothing is written in stone. You have the power to change anything you want to change.

Be patient and gentle with yourself. Being human has entitled all of us to a special inheritance. We have the right to make mistakes. Mistakes are part of living. Dwelling on our mistakes will not make them go away. Acknowledge them, learn from them and move on.

Love and be loved. We all have the capacity to love others and be loved. When you enjoy your uniqueness and importance in the fabric of life, and you accept who you are now and move creatively into the future, and you offer yourself the patience and gentleness of forgiveness – you are without a doubt loveable and you are capable of loving others.

The Mind-Body Connection

The liaison of mind and body creates harmony. Henry Droher in his book "The Immune Power Personality" suggests that we have key personality traits that boost our immune system. By developing the following traits we protect our health: recognition and acknowledgement of mind-body signals, a willingness to confide in others, the maintenance of a healthy lifestyle, a commitment to relationships and work, the ability to assert ourselves and an unselfish concern for the welfare of others.

Droher has not tapped into anything new. Yogis for thousands of years have acknowledged the importance of the relationship between the mind and the body to living a healthy physical, emotional and spiritual existence. Yoga and other similar practices help to develop a sense of balance and being centered in a hectic and often confusing world. This sense of being grounded allows us to get to know our own unique selves. In so doing clear choices for self improvement can be made.

Making a Change

The way you care for yourself says much about how you see yourself and how you want others to see you. It is your personal statement. An astute stranger can detect this message before you even have a

"The body's mischiefs, as Plato proves, proceed from the soul: and if the mind be not first satisfied the body can never be cured."

R O B E R T
B U R T O N

The Anatomy of

Melancholy

(1621)

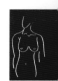

CHAPTER 17

chance to speak. First impressions are long lasting and may be difficult to alter, thus it is prudent to put your best foot forward from the very beginning.

The key to looking great is a healthy lifestyle. Taking steps to prevent problems from occurring, as well as maintaining a well-balanced program of diet and exercise, will ensure that your path through time is biologically smooth.

Although there is no true elixir of youth, there are certainly a great number of options to make you feel and look younger.

The most important factor is your internal beauty. Let it shine through. Enhancing your spiritual, emotional and intellectual growth will leave a legacy long after your body loses it's vitality.

Physical aging can be prevented to a certain degree, and the aged body can be rejuvenated. Take time to evaluate yourself by using the following steps:

Step 1:

Reflect upon the state of your general health – your diet, your habits, your exercise patterns, and the way you look. Using a full-length mirror, take a close look at your body, region by region. Take notes. Ask a friend, someone who is kind but honest. What hidden and visual imperfections should

you change? Are you willing to change? This should be a realistic self analysis.

Step 2:

Read the sections of this book that apply to you within the context of your honest self-evaluation. Write down all the options you feel may be potentially useful to you.

Step 3:

Evaluate each option independently. Look carefully at the risk-benefit ratios, at the costs, and at the potential physical or cosmetic disability. Cross out those options that weigh you down, but keep your list for future reference. Start with a list of 10 or fewer important items.

Step 4:

Put your list in order of priorities. What's most important to you now?

Step 5:

Carefully choose your doctor, dentist, and any other specialist you wish to consult. The title cosmetic or esthetic surgeon applies to a variety of surgical specialists who all have expertise in their specialties as well as in cosmetic surgery. Dermatologists, plastic surgeons, ophthalmologists, and otolaryngologists, play important roles in cosmetic surgery today.

 CHAPTER 17

Choosing a Cosmetic Surgeon

- You should feel comfortable and be able to discuss your problem openly with the specialist.

- Rely on your family, friends, family physician, or the regional medical association for a recommended specialist.

- Determine if a specialist is well trained and experienced by asking him or her for qualifications. Board certification in the United States and a Fellowship in Canada indicate that a physician has met the necessary requirements in a specialty. Further training in some highly specialized areas, such as laser surgery, is necessary for certain procedures. Most cosmetic surgeons will show you clinical photographs of their results. Ask about the number of procedures the physician has performed and his or her success rate. It is your body, and you have a right to know.

- Look for a physician who willingly discusses complications and risks, as well as benefits. Be wary of anyone who guarantees results. No credible practitioner will give guarantees. Also be wary of large assembly line surgical centers where personalized attention may be lost.

- Computer imaging is gaining popularity. It allows a patient the opportunity to see how they might look if a certain surgical procedure is done. This however is only an estimate, there is no way a computer can predict the out come of surgery. The results depend on the skill and experience of the surgeon, the equipment and technique being used, and the tissue response and unique healing capacity of the patient. Be wary of physicians who claim they can show you the outcome of a procedure prior to it being done. This is not possible.

Step 6:

Take into consideration the time you will need to take off from work if a cosmetic procedure is part of your plan. Your time commitment will vary from 1 day to 3 weeks, depending on the type of surgery to be performed.

There are also financial considerations. Cosmetic surgery is usually not covered by insurance plans and must be paid for by the patient.

Step 7:

Set the wheels in motion. Most people who undergo cosmetic procedures are pleased with the results. You should objectively examine your personal approach to the selected surgical options.

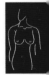

Results will probably disappoint you if you:

- are not sure whether you want surgery now or later;

- tend to be a perfectionist;

- are doing the procedure to please someone else;

- are expecting your body or face to look just like "this" or "that" or like someone else, such as a movie star or sports idol;

- have exceedingly high expectations;

- expect minimal or no post-operative pain or cosmetic disability;

- expect others to be as enthusiastic about the end results as you are.

Step 8:

Don't forget the total body image as it relates to cosmetics, hairstyle, dress, and the basics of good grooming. Be as cautious and critical in this area as in any; it is the finishing touch.

Enjoy a Fruitful Life

Once you have embarked on your personal program take time to enjoy the new you. Keep your mind open to change. As your body changes, you may want to adopt a new program for improvement. Above all be positive.

Cultural and societal influences are powerful and may or may not be healthy. Peoples desires for personal, physical, intellectual, psychological and emotional change are as complex and varied as are people themselves. Be sure that your desires for change are well founded and yours alone. You are your own person and your choices belong to you. The key to an exciting and fruitful life is you!

A P P E N D I X

The *Confessions* of a *Woman*

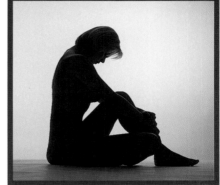

WHO

DECIDED

TO HAVE

LASER

RESURFACING

TO GET RID

OF THE

SIGNS

OF AGING

P A T I E N T   D I A R Y

DAY 1

I have not eaten since midnight and I'm hungry. I thought this would be difficult because I do not miss a meal unless absolutely necessary and it is! It, however, is absolutely necessary because I am having full face laser resurfacing under light sedation this afternoon.

"What for?" is not only the question everyone else asks me, but I also ask myself. I am 45 years old and the signs of aging and years in the sun when I was young without any protection have taken their toll. I not only have fine wrinkles but I have deep wrinkles around my eyes which are beginning to join to my smile lines, which I might add never go away after I have finished smiling! I have crosshatching under my eyes and my eyelids are beginning to droop. My lips appear permanently pursed from wrinkles that do not go away. Sounds frightful, doesn't it? Well it is not. I look quite normal for my age. But the lure of technology and the promise of a more youthful appearance have resulted in my decision to proceed.

For years I have been using the RetisolA and NeoStrata HQ combination and I think it has worked well to control the discoloration and texture changes that come with too much sun exposure over time. Then about 3 years ago I had a chemical peel. What an improvement - especially in color

and texture. Not so much in the wrinkles, which was a bit disappointing. After a chemical peel you look horrible for a number of days. The skin swells, crusts and peels. So I guess I am somewhat prepared for what to expect from laser resurfacing, although I am aware that I could be red for a long time after. It took my test site 3 months to fade.

I am thankful when they call me for surgery. It's now 3 o'clock and I am so hungry and thirsty. I haven't been able to drink anything for four hours. This is tough for a person who has trained themselves to drink 8 glasses of water a day.

I am a little anxious as Dr. Carle inserts the needle for the sedation and Dr. Groot takes pre-operative pictures. It's not too late to change my mind, but then again everyone is so friendly and reassuring. I know I am in competent hands.

In what seems like a flash I hear voices asking me how I am feeling and telling me it is all over. I know something is different because my face is burning and if feels a bit puffy. Part of me wants to get up but the other part just wants to stay there forever. The sedative has not quite worn off. I ask for a mirror.

My face is bright red, as though I had fallen asleep in the sun. In a way I guess a sunburn and laser resurfacing are similar in that they both are a form of photothermal (light/heat) damage to the skin. The difference is that the laser is more controlled and improves rather than damages the skin by stimulating the growth of new skin and realigning the collagen and elastins in the skin.

I go home and lie on the couch, my head elevated by big oversized pillows. Thank heavens for home delivery pizza because I am in no shape to cook and I am definitely hungry!

The only sign that the sedative is still in my system is that I occasionally trip over something or walk into the odd wall. Now I understand why you should not drive for 24 hours after the surgery.

The toughest part of the whole day was washing my face. When I splashed lukewarm water on it felt like I had shoved a thousand pins into it. I persisted because I know how important it is to keep the face clean. Then I applied Vaseline liberally (in big gobs) all over my face. Ouch! This really burned, but the discomfort subsided after a few minutes. Dr. Groot told me he uses a semi-occlusive dressing with some patients and just Vaseline with others. I think I would be claustrophobic under dressings.

After taking my antibiotics and anti-viral medication for cold sores, I propped my pillows, which I covered with old pillow cases, in an upright position and had a good sleep.

DAY 2

I woke up feeling like my face was a puff ball that was slowly simmering on the back burner. The image that greeted me in the mirror was a different person. Eyes sunk into swollen skin and a very red, gooey looking face. I had a shower, being sure not to let the water hit my face. I used damp gauze to gently cleanse my face (I haven't been brave enough to try soap yet), then reapplied Vaseline. Same burning sensation.

My face burned and throbbed all day. The Vaseline increases the intensity of the burning for a short time just after I apply it. A cold pack wrapped in a light cloth helped. To think that I had considered going in to work this morning! I am now beginning to think that I might not be able to go in to work for a while. Dr. Groot was not kidding when he told me to be prepared for a period of cosmetic disability.

I am not discouraged though because I have seen the results of people who have persevered. If I get half of the benefit they did I will be happy and think it all worthwhile.

In the meantime I have created a little nook for myself in the family room, surrounded by things to do. The portable telephone, books to read, cold packs for my face, Tylenol Extra-Strength,

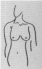

antibiotics, antiviral medications and lots of water to drink. With some pleasant background music playing I am sure I can sit this out for the next few days!

The burning persists throughout the day and my face continues to swell. Looking in the mirror is not a good idea. I really do not feel like getting up as moving seems to cause more discomfort to my face. If I could take Tylenol #3 I would, but unfortunately I can't have anything with codeine in it. Such is life. The Tylenol Extra-Strength helps a lot.

I used Neutrogena soap to clean my face today. My face was so gooey I had to do something. It was quite uncomfortable, but I felt much better afterwards. I have discovered that using cotton gauze to wash and cleanse my face is the best bet. They are very soft and gentle. I am also putting Telfa bandages on the sides of my face when I sleep at night, otherwise I am stuck to the pillow in the morning.

DAY 3

I soak my face for a long time before gently removing the Telfa bandages as I do not want to disturb the new skin. I continue to be very swollen, very red and very gooey, but the burning sensation has subsided a bit. My family is being very supportive and patient.

Once again I am in no mood or condition to venture forth into the world, but I feel like being up and around. I get busy doing the laundry and the dishes, as well as some things I never seem to have time for, like cleaning out drawers. By the afternoon I need to lie down and rest again.

The swelling continues to distort my face, but the red discoloration is beginning to take on a slightly brown tinge. As the oozing continues I find it necessary to gently clean my face with wet cotton gauze and reapply the Vaseline more frequently. If the ooze dries then it is really hard to remove. The Vaseline keeps my face from feeling tight, although the swelling makes it difficult to see or talk. The soft cotton gauze is also a godsend for blowing my nose. Kleenex is too harsh.

This is the day when the greatest patience is needed. Dr. Groot called to see how I was doing and to reassure me that all is going as expected. He told me that if the swelling persists he would give me a short course of cortisone to bring it under control.

DAY 4

Not much change in the morning, but as the day progresses the swelling begins to subside. By the end of the day I can look down and see my body rather than

YOUNG AS YOU LOOK

mounds of skin. By evening my facial features begin to return and there is some semblance of the old me in the mirror. A redder, gooier version I must add. I look like I have a birthmark that covers my whole face.

My face is really oozing today and I must constantly keep gently wiping it with wet gauze or it will become a really sticky mess. There is no doubt that proper care after this procedure is essential. I can see where a person could end up in a lot of trouble if infection sets in or if the temptation to pick is too great.

By evening a generalized crust has formed over my face - more so in areas where Dr. Groot went a bit deeper, such as under my eyes and along my upper lip. With this crust comes a very annoying itchiness. Dr. Groot told me that 20% of patients crust or scab and the rest just ooze but it doesn't make any difference in the outcome. Here again the Vaseline helps to soothe the skin and keep it supple so I can hold my desire to scratch in check.

DAY 5

The oozing seems to have stopped for the most part and my face is now crusty and itchy. On the advise of Dr. Groot I take an antihistamine to help relieve the itch. The swelling has almost all subsided, but the redness persists. I have opted not to go in to work

today. I thought I would be okay by now but I still look quite horrific. I guess I would equate the way I look to a person with a severe burn to the face. Even though I can see the progress, I think others would find it quite distressing to look at me.

The temptation to pick off the bits of skin that are pulling away from my face is very strong. Once again I use Vaseline as a means to control my urge. Dr. Groot assures me that it will take much longer to heal if I start picking and I really do not want to prolong this process nor do I want to cause a scar.

DAY 6

I am beginning to feel a bit house bound, so I decide to venture out to the bank. Big mistake. All the girls who know me well expressed great concern over my condition. They thought that I had somehow managed to stay in the sun far too long and have ended up with a very bad sunburn. I could not tell a lie, so I explained to them what I had done. They were all very intrigued and I found myself bombarded by all sorts of questions. I do not think they will ever look at me quite the same way again. I decide not to go grocery shopping as I had planned.

The scab like crusts are beginning to pull away, leaving red skin behind. I continue to apply Vaseline and resist the intense urge to pick, especially since the crusted areas are still quite itchy. I sometimes catch myself toying with the borders of the crusts. Each time I wash my face some of the crusts come off. Some areas are more resistant than others. Dr. Groot tells me that these are areas of deeper healing.

DAY 7

I am ready to have my life back and would dearly love to yank off the few remaining crusts. They are actually coming off quite quickly but I am still really anxious to be finished with this process. When Dr. Groot told me it would be 10 to 14 days before I would feel comfortable being in public I thought, "that's not so long". Now I realize that it is longer than I imagined.

However, I discipline myself and patiently wait for the crusts to come off on their own. There is no point in going through all this just to end up with a scar because I was not patient.

DAY 8

All the crusts are gone. The flakiness and redness persists. I tried to use a simple moisturizer rather than Vaseline but found I was still too dry and needed the heavy duty grease.

I am back into my routine of work and exercise. I use a thick cover-up makeup to tone down the redness. I am a bit self conscious about this but nobody seems to notice.

The best part of all is the obvious improvement in the texture and wrinkles on my face. There is no doubt that I look better. People who know what I have done comment in amazement on the change in my skin. They tell me I look younger. Great – that was definitely the goal! Dr. Groot said that he could touch-up around my eyes if I would like, but I am happy.

3 MONTHS LATER

My skin looks great. The flakiness did not last very long and I only used makeup for about 3 weeks. Then I felt comfortable with the bit of redness that remained. I have never worn foundation and was not comfortable using it all the time.

In my mind I look so much better than I did before. I would tend to use the word fresher rather than younger, although friends still comment that I definitely look younger.

About 6 weeks after the surgery I tried using the Retisol-A and NeoStrata HQ but I broke out in a rash. I have started using a very mild Stieva-A cream and will gradually build back up to the Retisol-A and NeoStrata HQ. I am also absolutely faithful about sunscreen, after all it was the sun that lead me to tell this story in the first place!

Glossary

A

ABSCESS: a localized pocket of pus.

ACETYLSALICYLIC ACID: a white crystalline compound that relieves pain and fever, but also causes thinning of the blood which can encourage bruising and bleeding. It is the generic name for aspirin.

ACNE (pimples): inflammation of the oil glands in the skin due to an oversensitivity to the normal level of hormones in the body.

AEROBICS: exercises, such as jogging, cycling, swimming, dance routines, and brisk walking, which increase the intake of oxygen.

AGE SPOTS: the layman's term for lentigos or seborrheic keratoses, benign brown growths on the skin that commonly appear with age.

AIDS: acronym for acquired immune deficiency syndrome, a virus induced illness that reduces the efficiency of the immune system to protect the body from disease.

ALLERGIC REACTIONS: a hyper-sensitivity to various environmental substances (allergens) that causes the body to respond in adverse ways. Symptoms may include a red, swollen rash on the skin or difficulty in breathing.

ALPHA HYDROXY ACID (AHA): a group of acids that reduce sun induced fine wrinkles and pigment spots by removing the superficial layers of the skin and drawing moisture into the tissue, causing the skin to fill out.

AMPOULES: sealed, glass or plastic containers that keep solutions sterile until required for injection.

ANDROGEN HORMONES: hormones that produce masculine characteristics in the body.

ANESTHETIC: a drug used to eliminate the sensation of pain. general a., the sensation of pain is removed throughout the body (commonly referred to as being put to sleep). local a., the sensation of pain is eliminated only in the area of the body where the anesthetic is administered.

ANTIOXIDANTS: substances, such as vitamins E and C, that prevent oxidation at the cellular level. It is surmised that oxidation is the chemical reaction central to the aging process.

AUGMENT: to increase or make larger, e.g., breast augmentation (enlargement of the breast).

BIOFEEDBACK: a technique used to voluntarily control involuntary movements or bodily processes.

B

B

BLEPHAROPLASTY (eyelid lift): a surgical procedure that corrects baggy eyelids by removing excess skin and fat from the upper and lower eyelids and tightens up lax muscles around the eyes.

BRIDGE: a dental device that fills in gaps from missing teeth; fixed bridge, a permanent bridge; removable bridge, a bridge that can be put in and taken out of the mouth.

BRUXISM: grinding of the teeth at times other than chewing, especially when sleeping.

C

CANNULA: a hollow rigid or flexible surgical tube, which is rigid or flexible depending on its use.

CAPSULAR CONTRACTURE: a layer of fibrous tissue that encapsulates a breast implant causing the breast to feel unnaturally hard.

CAPSULOTOMY: the process of breaking down the fibrous or scar tissue of a capsular contracture of a breast implant; closed capsulotomy, the fibrous tissue is fractured by compressing the breast from the outside; open capsulotomy, the scar tissue that has enclosed the implant is partially removed through the original surgical incision.

CELLULITE: irregular contours of fat over the buttocks, hips, and thighs, which make the skin look dimpled.

CHEMICAL PEEL: a resurfacing technique in which one of a variety of chemical agents is applied to the skin to remove its superficial layers. In so doing, the skin is regenerated and rejuvenated through the removal of wrinkles, the smoothing of irregular pigmentation, and the growth of new skin.

CHERRY ANGIOMAS: bright red, benign blood vessel tumors of the skin that range in size from a pin prick to the size of a drop of water.

CHOLESTEROL: a steroid alcohol found in a variety of foods which, if consumed in excessive amounts, is thought to contribute to the blocking of the arteries (arteriosclerosis) and can leave deposits in the skin in the form of yellow bumps.

COLD SORE: a blister arising from the herpes simplex virus.

COLLAGEN: the principal supporting protein of the skin, bones, cartilage, and connective tissue of the body.

COMPOSITE BONDING: the process of adhering a plastic-like material to teeth to improve their appearance.

CORTISONE: a hormone used to control inflammation.

COSMETIC SURGEON: a general term referring to a physician with special training, skills, and interest in one or more surgical techniques to improve the cosmetic appearance of an individual. Plastic surgeons and dermatologists are most commonly categorized as cosmetic surgeons, although some ophthalmologists and otolaryngologists may also have

YOUNG AS YOU LOOK

training in cosmetic procedures related to their specialties.

CROW'S FEET: wrinkles that spread out from the corners of the eyes.

CROWN: a porcelain or porcelain-bonded-to-gold covering applied over the entire surface of the tooth.

CRYOTHERAPY: a dermatologic therapy that uses a cooling agent, such as liquid nitrogen or solid carbon dioxide (dry ice), for a variety of treatments.

D

DANDRUFF: a dry, scaly condition of the skin on the scalp and, less often, on the face and the torso.

DEHYDRATE: the removal of water or moisture.

DEPILATORIES: hair removal agents that dissolve unwanted hair.

DERMABRASION: a resurfacing technique that removes the superficial layers of the skin enabling new, rejuvenated skin to replace scarred, wrinkled, and irregularly pigmented skin utilizing a whirling bit to remove the superficial layers of skin.

DERMATOLOGIST: a medical doctor who specializes in diseases and disorders of the skin.

DERMIS: the second layer of the skin, which contains elastins (elastic protein) to provide skin tone and suppleness; collagen (architectural protein) for strength and structure; blood vessels for the delivery of essential nutrients and the removal of wastes; nerves, making the skin one of the most sensitive organs in the body; oil glands to lubricate the skin; and sweat glands to regulate fluctuations in body temperature.

DIHYDROXYACETONE (DHA): the active agent in tanning creams which reacts with the top layer of the skin through oxidation to produce a natural golden hue.

DILATE: to increase in size beyond normal dimensions.

E

EDEMA: abnormally large amounts of fluid between the cells of body tissue.

ELASTIN: elastic tissue in the second layer of the skin that provides skin tone and suppleness.

ELECTRODESICCATION: the process of removing small skin problems such as milia, cherry angiomas, and minute veins with an electric current transferred through a needle.

ELECTROLYSIS: a procedure to remove unwanted hair by passing an electric current into a hair follicle, rendering it inactive, and causing the hair to fall out.

ENDORPHINS: natural opiates released by the brain during prolonged exercise and thought to be responsible for a self-induced feelings of well being.

ENKEPHALINES: natural opiates released by the brain during prolonged exercise and thought to be responsible for a self induced feelings of well being.

E **EPIDERMIS:** the protective top layer of the skin where pigment cells, which give color to the skin, are found.

ESTHETIC: pertaining to beauty; artistic; pleasing to the eye.

F **FACE LIFT:** a surgical procedure designed to correct three problems in the lower half of the face: poor muscle tone, causing laxity in the neck and cheek areas; too much fat in the jowl, chin, and neck regions; and excess amounts of skin in the lower half of the face, causing wrinkles.

FIBROCYSTIC DISEASE: a condition where a cystic space develops in the glandular tissue of the breast and is overgrown with fibrous tissue.

FIBROUS: composed of fibers.

FOOD AND DRUG ADMINISTRATION (FDA): a regulatory body of the United States government responsible for the quality and safety of foods and drugs.

FREE RADICALS: chemical agents that contribute to the wear and tear on cells through a chemical reaction known as oxidation and thought to be central to the aging process.

G **GRANULOMA:** a hard bump caused by the body's cells walling off foreign material.

H **HAIR FOLLICLE:** part of a strand of hair that is alive and below the surface of the skin.

HAIR SHAFT: the dead, yet visible, portion of a strand of hair.

HAIR TRANSPLANT: a surgical procedure to remove hair from a donor site, usually on the back of the head, and transfer it to a recipient site, usually on the crown or top of the head.

HEALTH PROTECTION BRANCH (HPB): a regulatory body of Health and Welfare Canada that is responsible for the safety and quality of foods and drugs.

HEMATOMA: a tumor-like collection of blood in a localized area.

HEMOGLOBIN: red cells of the blood that carry oxygen.

HEPATITIS: inflammation of the liver, commonly caused by a viral infection.

HERPES SIMPLEX: an acute viral infection that causes watery blisters, frequently referred to as cold sores, on the skin and mucus membranes.

HUMAN ADJUVANT DISEASE (HAD): a broad term encompassing a variety of autoimmune disease states including rheumatoid arthritis, dermatomyositis and lupus erythematosus.

HYPERPIGMENTATION: a condition where one area of the skin produces more melanin making it darker than the surrounding skin.

Y O U N G   A S   Y O U   L O O K

HYPOPIGMENTATION: a condition where the pigment cells produce inadequate amounts of melanin resulting in a localized area of skin being lighter than normal.

IMMUNE SYSTEM: a system within the body that protects it from disease and infection.

IMPLANTS: organic or inorganic material inserted or grafted into a predetermined part of the body.

INFLAMMATION: a condition where the body tissue reacts to injury with swelling, redness, pain, and heat.

INFRAMAMMARY FOLD: the fold under the breast where the skin of the breast meets the skin of the chest wall

INGEST: the act of taking food or medicine into the body by mouth.

INTRAVENOUS: within a vein or veins.

IRRITATION: a state of undue sensitivity.

LANGERHANS CELLS: star-shaped cells found deep in the epidermis which recognize disease and other threats to the body and which subsequently mobilize the white blood cells to protect against intruders.

LASABRASION: resurfacing of the skin with a surgical laser by vaporizing away the superficial layers of the epidermis and dermis so new skin, free of fine wrinkles and pigment changes, will grow.

LASER: an acronym for light amplification by stimulated emission of radiation. Laser frequently refers to a group of instruments that produce a pure monochromatic light. The purpose of the instrument varies depending on the type of light emitted.

LENTIGO: a benign, brown spot on the skin caused by a localized increase in the production of melanin. It is usually associated with aging.

LIPOSUCTION: a procedure where fat is suctioned from localized areas of the body.

LUPUS ERYTHEMATOSUS: a condition which can affect the skin and the internal organs where the body makes an error in recognizing its own tissue and falsely perceives it as foreign thereby attacking itself with an immunologic reaction.

MALAR BAGS: baggy skin that appears at the junction of the lower eyelids and upper part of the cheek bones.

MALE PATTERN HAIR LOSS: a hereditary predisposition for the loss of hair on the head.

MAMMOGRAPHY: an x-ray of the soft tissue of the breast.

MELANIN: a dark pigment found in the skin, hair, choroid coat of the eye, and part of the brain.

I

L

M

M

METABOLIC RATE: the speed at which metabolism takes place.

METABOLISM: the process of transforming food to supply energy to the body.

MICROLIPID: small amounts of fat; microlipid transfer, a procedure whereby small amounts of fat are taken from one part of the body and injected into another.

MILIA: tiny, oil gland cysts in the skin.

MINOXIDIL: a medication that helps to control high blood pressure when taken in tablet form and encourages hair growth when applied to the skin.

N

NAIL PLATE: the hard, flat, translucent, and visible surface of the nail.

NECROSIS: pertaining to the death of tissue, usually in small, localized areas.

O

OPHTHALMOLOGIST: a medical doctor who is an eye specialist.

ORTHODONTIST: a dentist who specializes in the realignment of the teeth so that the bite is functional and esthetically pleasing.

ORTHOGNATHIC SURGERY: surgery which corrects the jaw bones when they are positioned in such a

way as to cause facial disharmony and dental dysfunction.

OTOLARYNGOLOGIST: a medical doctor who is an ear, nose, and throat specialist.

OXIDATION: a chemical change that occurs in tissue when it combines with oxygen.

P

PERI-AREOLAR: around the nipple of the breast.

PERIODONTAL DISEASE: disease of the gums caused by bacteria growing on the teeth.

PIGMENT: natural coloring of the skin.

PLASTIC SURGEON: a medical doctor who specializes in reconstructive and cosmetic surgery.

PRECANCERS: benign spots on the skin which tend to develop into cancers.

PROFILOPLASTY: a common medical term for the alteration of the structural proportions that determine the profile, for example, the nose and the chin.

PSORALEN: a chemical agent that stimulates pigment cells to produce more melanin when exposed to the sun. It is found in tan accelerators.

PULSE DYE LASER: a laser system that produces a target specific light causing selective destruction of small blood vessels with accompanying bruising. This laser removes portwine hemangionas and cutaseous vascular lesions from the skin.

PUNCH TRANSPLANT: a procedure that transfers a circular piece of skin from a donor area, usually behind the ear, to a recipient area, usually on the face, to replace damaged or scarred skin.

R **RADIATION:** light rays emitted from the sun in the form of ultraviolet A, ultraviolet B, and ultraviolet C spectrums.

RESURFACING: a procedure to alter the top layer of the skin through chemical or mechanical means.

RHINOPLASTY: surgery that alters the shape or structure of the nose.

ROOT CANAL: a procedure that removes the blood vessels and nerves in the root of the tooth.

S **SCLERA:** the white portion of the eye; scleral show, when the white portion of the eye below the iris is visible.

SCLEROTHERAPY: a technique whereby a solution of concentrated salt, sugar, and alcohol or other agents is injected into veins. This irritates the lining of the veins causing them to adhere together and to subsequently shrink and disappear.

SEBORRHEA (seborrheic dermatitis):

dandruff that has caused inflammation.

SEBORRHEIC KERATOSIS (age spots, liver spots): benign, brown spots on the skin that occur with aging.

SEDATION: the process of creating calm, especially through medication.

SEROMA: a tumor-like collection of fluid in a localized area.

SERUM: the clear component of blood.

SILASTIC: a plastic-like material used in certain types of implants.

SILICONE: an inorganic material, made up of a compound containing the element silicon and used for a variety of implants.

SKIN CANCER: a cellular tumor of the skin that is defined according to the cells of the skin involved. Squamous cell cancer, basal cell cancer, and melanomas are three of the most common skin cancers.

SKIN TAGS: superfluous stubs of skin that develop when the skin is confused as to which direction to grow, so it simply grows outward. They may occur anywhere on the body.

SOFT LASER: cool beam, nonsurgical laser lights that are thought to cause mild inflammation and edema of the superficial layers of the skin to temporarily puff up fine wrinkles. Other photochemical skin reactions may occur but have not been scientifically proven.

S

SPIDER VEINS: dilated blood vessels, in particular, small, superficial, dilated veins on the legs.

STRETCH MARKS: lines of stretched skin which develop when the skin's building blocks (collagen and elastin) cannot keep up with its need for growth. Medically referred to as striae.

STRIAE: see stretch marks.

SUBCUTANEOUS: below the first two layers of skin.

SUBGLANDULAR: below glandular tissue; for example, of the breast.

SUBMUSCULAR: below underlying muscle; for example, of the breast.

SUCTION LIPOLYSIS: see liposuction.

SUN PROTECTION FACTOR (SPF): the factor for the amount of time greater than normal that it takes ultraviolet light to burn the skin.

SWEAT RASH: layman's term for miliaria, which are small, red bumps on the skin caused by sweat retention.

T

TAN ACCELERATORS: an agent that speeds up the natural tanning process or production of melanin in the skin, lowering the sun exposure time needed for a desired tan.

TANNING BEDS: beds of light bulbs that usually emit ultraviolet A rays to artificially induce a sun tan.

TANNING CREAMS: creams containing dihydroxyacetone (DHA) that react with the top layer of the skin through oxidation to produce a natural, golden hue.

TELANGIECTASIA: small, superficial, dilated veins on the face, neck, and chest.

TEMPOROMANDIBULAR JOINT: the point at which the jaw bone or mandible comes into contact with the skull or temporal bone.

TOPICAL: on the skin.

TOXIC: caused by or acting as a poison.

TOXIN: a poisonous agent.

TRANSAXILLARY: through the armpit.

TRETINOIN: a topical agent that has proven to be effective in the treatment of acne, fine wrinkles, irregular pigment, and texture changes of the skin. Also known generically as retinoic acid and by the trade names Stieva-A, Retin-A, Vitamin A Acid, Rejuva-A, Renova and Retisol-A.

TUMMY TUCK: a surgical procedure that improves the esthetic appearance of an abdomen which has an excess amount of skin with stretch marks, too much fat, and a loss of muscle tone in the abdominal region.

TUMESCENT LIPOSUCTION: a type of suction lipolysis in which the fat compartment is initially expanded with a dilute local anesthetic solution.

YOUNG AS YOU LOOK

TYROSINE: an amino acid (protein component) that contributes to the production of melanin.

ULTRASONIC LIPOSUCTION: a method of liposuction where sound waves are passed along a cannula causing emulsification of the fat prior to aspiration.

U

ULTRAVIOLET: invisible light rays emitted by the sun that are just beyond the visible spectrum.

ULTRAVIOLET-A RAYS (UVA rays): the longest ultraviolet light rays emitted by the sun, causing damage to the epidermis and the dermis of the skin and to the eyes over long periods of exposure.

ULTRAVIOLET-B RAYS (UVB rays): the mid-length ultraviolet light rays emitted by the sun, causing damage to the epidermis and the dermis of the skin and which may also be harmful to the eyes.

ULTRAVIOLET-C RAYS (UVC rays): the shortest ultraviolet light rays emitted by the sun. If these rays were not absorbed by the ozone layer they would cause severe bodily harm.

UREA: a chemical that draws moisture into tissues of the skin.

VARIABLE PULSE WIDTH LASER: a laser system with the capacity to alter the time application of light impact on blood vessels. It is used to remove red vascular lesions from the skin without bruising.

VARICOSE VEINS: large, dilated veins of the legs.

VENEER: a resin or porcelain facing that is placed over the surface of the tooth to improve the appearance of the teeth.

V

XANTHINES: a group of stimulants, including theobromine and caffeine, that may be found in chocolate, coffee, and tea causing dilation of blood vessels and stimulation of the muscles, especially the heart.

X

Index

B

birthmark(s)   16, 105, 281

blackheads   12, 38, 48,

bleaching   53, 55, 197

bleaching cream   19, 197, 257, 259

blepharoplasty   141–146, 148–149, 284

blood vessels   8-10, 105-106, 135, 255-257

blush   46

body analysis   264

bonding (see composite bonding) 284

Botox (see botulinum exotoxin)   102, 143, 149

botulinum exotoxin (see Botox)   102, 143, 149

braces   180, 188

breast(s)   18–19, 22, 210–230

breast augmentation   211, 216, 218, 220–221, 227, 229, 267

breast asymmetry   217, 225, 229

breast cancer   212, 220, 226

breast feeding   210, 218, 222, 224, 227, 229–230

breast implants   210

breast lift   211, 222, 227–229

breast reconstruction   211, 213

breast reduction   211, 221–222, 225, 228–229, 267

bridge   186–187, 284

brow lift   15, 137, 146–147, 149–153

bruising   136, 144–146, 148, 151, 215, 223, 226, 228, 233, 235, 237, 245–246, 249–250, 256

brushing (see teeth)   182

bruxism   185, 284

bulimia   236

buttocks   18, 22, 79, 232, 242–243, 253

C

calcium   38, 72–74

Calmurid (see chemically enhanced moisturizers)   260

caloric restrictions   75

camouflage   45, 133, 139, 145–146, 151–153, 194, 197, 199, 205, 207–208, 218, 257, 260, 266–267

cancer   8, 29, 212, 220, 229

cannula   130, 135, 233, 235, 245–246, 248, 251, 284

capping (see crowns)   184

capsular contracture   217–218, 284

capsulotomy   284

carbon dioxide laser (see CO_2 laser) 18, 104, 111–112, 138, 143–145, 148, 151–152, 253–259

cellulite   18, 242, 249, 252–253, 284

Cetaphil lotion   40

cheeks   15, 30, 132, 156, 164–5, 167, 243

cheek implants   164–165

chemical depilatories   136, 194, 197,

chemical peel   14, 33, 49–50, 110–111, 121–123, 125–127, 137, 143, 147, 260, 284

chemically enhanced moisturizers   44, 60, 260–261

chemotherapy   55

cherry angioma   125, 230, 284

chin   14, 45–46, 135, 156, 160–164, 189,

chin implants   161–162

cholesterol   284

chronic fatigue syndrome   212

chronological age   9–10, 146, 149,

cleanser(s)   37–40

cleansing creams   39–40

clothing   264–270

CO_2 laser (see carbon dioxide laser) 104, 111–112, 143–145, 148,

cold sore (see herpes)   114, 118, 120, 196, 279, 284

E

eye makeup 47
eyebrow(s) 45, 47, 49, 138, 141, 149, 197
eyelid lift (see blepharoplasty) 15, 17, 137, 141–142
eyelid plasty (see eyelid lift and blepharoplasty) 142
eyes 13, 15, 141, 171–178

F

fabric 15, 18,
facelift 15, 17, 132–148, 265–268, 286
facial harmony 155–167
facial surgery 132–153
facial veins (see telangiectasia) 16, 105, 125
facials 48–49, 137
farsighted 47, 170, 172–173, 175–176
fashion 3, 264–270
fat layer 8, 36
fat necrosis 224–225
fat pads 13, 143–144, 148, 242
fat redistribution (see microlipid transfers) 15
feet 258–259
Fibrel implants 95–97
fibrocystic disease 226, 229, 286
fibrous protein (see collagens) 9, 12,
finasteride (see Propecia , Proscar) 201
fitness 65–81
flap graft (see hair transplanting) 203
flossing 181
flutamide (see Euflex) 198
Food and Drug Administration (FDA) 36, 42, 195, 201, 286
foundations 46
freckled 10, 108
Fucidin 197, 257

G

gels 25, 58, 86, 97, 195
gigantomastia 226
glycolic acid 42–44, 91–92, 259
gravity 13–14, 17, 132, 141, 149, 152, 221, 227
gums 180–182, 187–188

H

hair 52–58, 133–134, 194–208
hair care products 56–58
hair follicle 52, 55, 195–197, 199, 201, 286
hair loss 54–57, 194, 199–208
hair piece 207–208
hair root 10, 52, 55, 199
hair shaft 52, 196 , 286
hair spray 58, 203
hair transplant 4, 201–207, 286
hair weaving 207–208
hands 258–261
heart 67, 201, 207, 261
Health Protection Branch (HPB) 36, 42, 286
hemangioma 105
hematoma 138–139, 147–148, 152, 216–218, 224, 239, 248, 286
hepatitis 244
heredity 9, 13–14, 16, 18–19, 199, 252, 258
herpes (see coldsore) 19, 196, 286
hormonal imbalance 8, 197hormones 10–11, 16, 34, 42, 44, 198–199, 201, 219, 252
human adjuvant disease (HAD) 211–213, 217, 286
Hylaform 93–98
hydroquinone 89, 91, 148, 259
hyperpigmentation 45,115, 120, 197, 223, 286
hypopigmentation 47, 120, 287

S

T

About the Authors

DON GROOT
M.D.,F.R.C.P.(Canada), F.A.C.P. (U.S.A.)

Don Groot is one of North America's foremost authorities on cosmetic laser surgery and the impact of aging on the skin. He holds fellowships in dermatology and laser surgery in both Canada and the United States. In addition to his own thriving dermatologic surgery center, Dr. Groot is an Associate Clinical Professor at the University of Alberta's Department of Medicine. He has published numerous scientific papers, contributed chapters to several medical textbooks, served as Editor-in-Chief of the Journal of Contemporary Dermatology, hosted seminars, and moderated television and radio programs. He is best known for his expertise in cosmetic dermatology and laser surgery. From San Francisco to Istanbul, London to Brasilia, Barcelona to Sydney he has taught plastic surgeons and dermatologists his surgical techniques.

Dr. Groot has for the last decade acted as a team physician for a professional hockey club in the National Hockey League and personally participates in community games of hockey and basketball. He shares his love for flying an old Cessna, astronomy, fly fishing and mountain sports with his family who divide their recreational time between Vancouver Island and the Canadian Rockies.

PATRICIA JOHNSTON
M.Cl.Sc., M.B.A.

Patricia Johnston holds advanced degrees in clinical science and business administration. As the president of InForum, she publishes and produces medical information and is a columnist for a local magazine on women's issues. She has published many scientific articles, co-authored the chapters of several medical textbooks and has acted as a research associate on several dermatologic projects. As a lecturer she has been in demand from New Orleans to London and from San Francisco to Frankfurt. As a business consultant she works with physicians to create practises which meet their needs and the needs of their patients.

Ms. Johnston is an enthusiastic student of yoga and water color painting. Her love of the out-of-doors takes her to the Canadian Rockies and Vancouver Island where she enjoys running, hiking, mountain biking, canoeing, kayaking, sailing and skiing with Don Groot and their two sons.

Order Form

If you wish to order more copies of the **Young As You Look** book or video, please mail or fax the following form to InForum:

InForum
207, 11523 - 100 Avenue
Edmonton, Alberta
Canada. T5K 0J8

Phone: (403) 488-6809
Fax: (403) 482-7097

Web Site: www.drgroot.ca

PRICE

_____@ $19.95 US or $24.95 CAN per video = _____

_____@ $19.95 US or $24.95 CAN per book = _____

_____@ $4.00 Shipping = _____

_____TOTAL = _____

METHOD OF PAYMENT

❑ Cheque   ❑ Money Order   ❑ Visa   ❑ MasterCard

Credit Card No. _____

Expiry Date _____

Day Time Telephone _____

Cardholder's Signature _____

Cardholder's Name (Please Print)_____

Ship To: _____

_____

_____

_____